CANCER, TRAUMA & EMOTIONS

A TRADITIONAL MEDICINE PATH TO SPIRITUAL WHOLENESS

Brandon LaGreca, LAc, MAcOM

Foreword by

Matt Mumber, MD

EMPOWERED PATIENT PRESS

CANCER, TRAUMA & EMOTIONS:
A Traditional Medicine Path to Spiritual Wholeness

Copyright © 2024 Brandon LaGreca
eBook ISBN: 978-1-7329996-6-4
Paperback ISBN: 978-1-7329996-7-1
Hardcover ISBN: 978-1-7329996-8-8

Cover design: Jess Estrella
Author photograph: Carla Gesell

Medical disclaimer: This book is intended to supplement but not replace the advice of a trained health professional. If you know or suspect you have a health problem, you should consult a health professional. All efforts have been made to ensure the accuracy of the information contained in this book as of publication. The author specifically disclaims any liability, loss, or risk, personal or otherwise, that is incurred as a direct or indirect consequence of the use and application of any of the contents of this book.

For Wild & Wooly

 споль

"You gotta resurrect the deep pain within you and give it
a place to live that's not within your body.
Let it live in art. Let it live in writing. Let it live in
music. Let it be devoured by building brighter connections.
Your body is not a coffin for pain to be buried in.
Put it somewhere else."

—Ehime Ora

CONTENTS

FOREWORD

As a radiation oncologist with a deep commitment to integrative medicine, I have long been fascinated by the complex interplay between mind, body, and spirit in the face of life-threatening illness. In my work with cancer patients, I have witnessed firsthand how unresolved emotional wounds profoundly impact physical health and healing. It is within this framework that Brandon LaGreca's latest book, *Cancer, Trauma & Emotions: A Traditional Medicine Path to Spiritual Wholeness*, finds its profound relevance.

As a conventional oncologist, I was trained to focus primarily on the physical aspects of cancer: histology and location of the primary tumor, the stage of disease, the optimal antineoplastic treatment protocols. My work in integrative oncology reveals that fixing is not the same as healing. To approach the difficult work of healing requires a much broader perspective. Cancer is both a physical disturbance and a systemic imbalance that affects the entire being—body, mind, and spirit—as they are experienced through the lens of self, culture, and the natural world.

In my own practice, I have seen how integrative approaches can transform the cancer care experience. Patients who engage in practices that address their mental, emotional and spiritual needs often exhibit greater resilience, improved quality of life, and, in some cases, better clinical outcomes. Brandon's work aligns with this integrative philosophy, offering a comprehensive approach that honors the complexity of the human experience.

Brandon is a cancer survivor, licensed acupuncturist, and practitioner of traditional Chinese medicine. He takes us on a journey to the frontiers of mind-body medicine, weaving together cutting-edge science with the ancient wisdom of traditional Chinese medicine. Drawing on the latest research in fields like epigenetics, neuroscience, and psychoneuroimmunology, Brandon reveals how trauma alters the terrain of the body, creating a fertile ground for disease to take root. He explores the surprising connections between adverse childhood experiences, learned helplessness, and the "Type C" personality, showing how unresolved emotional pain may manifest as cancer and other chronic conditions.

This book is not just about the science of how we get sick—it's about the art of how we can stay well and how we can approach healing. Brandon illuminates the power of the mind-body-spirit connection and provides a wealth of practical tools for working with emotions, beliefs, and energy to support the healing process. He draws on a wide range of modalities, from cognitive to somatic therapies, offering a practical roadmap for releasing the past, restoring resilience, and reclaiming wholeness.

One of the strengths of Brandon's approach is his emphasis on the "Heart-mind," the spiritual essence of each individual that transcends the purely physical realm. In traditional Chinese medicine, the Heart is seen as the emperor of the body, governing our thoughts, emotions, and overall well-being. By tapping into this innate wisdom and cultivating a state of coherence between the Heart-mind and body, we can access a profound source of healing.

Another important theme of the book is the role of community in healing. Brandon emphasizes the importance of social support, connection, and belonging in promoting resilience and well-being. As a medical professional, I have seen how the love and care of family, friends, and community can make all the difference in a patient's healing journey. *Cancer, Trauma & Emotions* reminds us that we are not meant to face life's challenges alone and that the power of human connection can be a profound, foundational resource.

Ultimately, what makes *Cancer, Trauma & Emotions* such an important and timely book is its message of hope and empowerment. Brandon reminds us that even in the face of life's greatest challenges, we have the capacity to heal, to grow, and to transform. By working with the mind-body-spirit connection, we can tap into a deep well of resilience and inner strength, finding meaning and purpose in the midst of adversity.

Whether you are a cancer patient seeking to support your own journey, a clinician looking to expand your tool kit, or simply a seeker on the path of personal growth and transformation, this book has something to offer.

I encourage you to approach this book with an open mind and a compassionate heart. Allow yourself to be touched by the stories, the insights, and the practices that Brandon shares. And most importantly, trust in your own inner wisdom and your innate capacity to heal. For as Brandon so eloquently reminds us, the journey to wholeness is not about becoming someone else, but about remembering who we truly are.

Matt Mumber, MD
Radiation Oncologist and Integrative Medicine Practitioner
Editor, *Integrative Oncology: Principles and Practice*
Co-author of *Sustainable Wellness: An Integrative Approach to Transform Your Mind, Body, and Spirit*

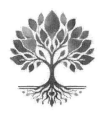

INTRODUCTION

Arianne was 34 when she was diagnosed with stage 3 lipo-sar-coma. A successful doctor of physical therapy with a newfound passion and certification in kettlebell training, Arianne was the model of health. Then an unusual pinch in her calf, followed by a palpable mass behind her knee, led to an MRI and biopsy that began Arianne's personal cancer journey. It was just a few months before her wedding.

I say "personal" cancer journey because Arianne was no strang-er to the trauma that is cancer. Years earlier, her brother Dave died from cancer after his third bout. Yet Arianne's experience of trauma goes back even further, being a victim of rape as a teenager. Arianne bares her soul in her memoir, *Rise Up*, where she shares the des-peration and numbness of being sexually violated.

"I didn't want to interact with anyone," she writes. "I didn't want to look at anyone or have anyone look at me. I just wanted to get away."

Later in her career, but before her cancer diagnosis, Arianne suffered from hip and pelvis pain. Although skilled in physical medicine, she had a keen sense that clear structural issues, such as a bilateral labral tear in her case, can become recalcitrant problems complicated by one's inner life. In her own words:

> I realize in hindsight that there may have been some emotional pain stored in there, too. There were so many things that had happened in my life that I didn't deal with entirely. Knowing what I know now, those emotions are stored in our bodies, specifically in our fascial tissue. So, although my pain could be reproduced with movement, otherwise known as mechanical pain, I realize how heavily my emotional experience impacted my physical pain.

Fast forward to her cancer diagnosis. Arianne underwent aggressive conventional oncology treatment: chemotherapy, proton radiation therapy, and surgery. With a promising career ahead of her and months away from marrying the love of her life, Arianne had to find the power within to rise up.

How could someone who is the embodiment of health receive such a dire diagnosis? And how might Arianne's history of trauma and her fears and beliefs about cancer, after witnessing her brother's struggle, relate to her illness?

Merriam-Webster defines trauma as "a disordered psychic or behavioral state resulting from severe mental or emotional stress or physical injury." Likewise, cancer is "a malignant tumor of potentially unlimited growth that expands locally by invasion and systemically by metastasis." The former is a disease of the mind, while the latter is a disease of the body.

After much reflection, I have concluded that trauma and cancer carry the same definition: a wound that isn't healing. At first blush, this definition will seem absurd to the Western reductionist mind, but it makes sense if you suspend the brain's attempt to categorize and delineate cancer cell types and the activity of oncogenes. That world exists, but it has not yet produced the stunning cures in conventional oncology that we all hope for. We need to change our thinking about the problem of cancer to be analogous to how we think about the origins of and healing from a traumatic experience.

Bridging the experience of trauma to the condition of cancer requires us to look beyond the artificial divide between the thoughts we think, the emotions we feel, and our physical health. This brings us to the central thesis of this book—that the governing influence of well-being lies in leading from heart-centered consciousness, a notion I and others call the Heart-mind.

In subsequent chapters, we will delve into the science and wisdom traditions that posit a heart-centered rather than brain-centered consciousness is the driver of human experience. While that dichotomy might seem semantical, shifting our understanding of awareness to include the feeling body and spiritual Heart in addition to the thinking brain has important implications for how we heal. This approach changes our directive in medicine to restoring wholeness rather than treating individual maladies.

While seeking a cure is the obvious goal of someone diagnosed with cancer, healing invites us to become more empowered through the process. This underscores how healing from cancer and trauma flow in the same stream. Ideally, we realize a plan to both cure and heal from cancer. But while the former takes treatment, the latter requires awareness, introspection, and a willingness to swim in the psychospiritual undercurrent of disease.

Consider how Western culture, and by extension the conventional medical system, establishes norms of treatment. If an individual is injured in a motor vehicle accident, an X-ray can diagnose a fracture in the sternum or surrounding ribs. If the injury is severe, the emergency room physician may rush the patient into surgery. Justifiably, the situation necessitates an immediate response. Hospitals are designed to efficiently triage such trauma.

Now consider a patient with shortness of breath and chest pain. It wouldn't take long for a workup by a cardiologist to diagnose angina pectoris and prescribe the appropriate treatment. Here, too, conventional medicine is equipped with blood tests, electrocardiograms, and catheterization procedures to identify and ameliorate the disease process. Although not an acute physical trauma, the mechanism underlying the physiological imbalance is well recognized.

Finally, consider an individual who is despondent following emotional heartbreak. Bloodwork may be normal, and diagnostic tests would not reveal a physiological imbalance that correlates with the deep grief of loss. Yet the person's experience of emotional pain could be as debilitating as any physical pain. Unless an individual is threatening harm to oneself or others, treatment may not be prioritized. A psychiatrist may prescribe an antidepressant after a brief consultation, and the patient may have to wait a few weeks for an appointment with a therapist. Acknowledgement of the severity of emotional trauma is not met with the same immediacy as physical trauma.

This is not a criticism of modern psychotherapy. I'm sure many psychologists are frustrated with not being more integrated into mainstream healthcare and lacking adequate reimbursement from health insurance. This frustration is shared with many providers of integrative medicine.

What underlies this imbalance in treatment priorities? I've pondered this question over the years and have precious few insights. One possibility is the historical conditioning to view the human frame as a machine, prioritizing physical medicine. This notion rose to prominence in the modern world and has only become more ingrained in the information age. We are a citizenry specialized in tasks due to the division of labor; most members of the working class are no longer peasant farmers tied to the rhythms of nature.

There is nothing inherently wrong with a high degree of advancement in physical medicine, as anyone who has experienced a physical trauma will attest when lifesaving medicine is applied. The problem lies in having the buck stop there—literally and metaphorically. Funding for biomedical research is heavily skewed toward pharmaceutical development and new procedures. This suggests a philosophical divide. Conventional medicine prefers to study that which can be neatly categorized. Emotional trauma is messy, nuanced, and requires a holistic approach to wellness. It entails a philosophical shift from the disease affecting the person to a focus on the person experiencing the disease.

This divide has long accompanied the practice of medicine and shows up in our understanding of the origins and treatment of cancer and trauma. When a cancer patient consults with me, I make clear at the onset that the patient's oncologist is the disease expert, while my role is to be the health expert. Conventional oncology is a highly refined science of tissue biopsies and genetic testing. By contrast, traditional, holistic medicine is unparalleled in restoring wellness and reinforcing resilience. Together, these paradigms frame an integrative model that can address the disease while strengthening the body, mind, and spirit to optimize outcomes.

Drawing from my education in traditional Chinese medicine (TCM) and clinical practice as a licensed acupuncturist, the dominant paradigm of this book's portrayal of holistic medicine stems from Eastern thinking. Yet Western philosophy also has roots in a model of medicine that is equally focused on generating health as on eliminating disease.

The Greek god of medicine is Asclepius, whose staff picto-graphically composes the image seen in the logo of many modern clinics and hospitals. Asclepius mythologically represents the heal-ing arts. The counterpoint to this mode of medicine is Asclepius's daughter Hygieia, from whose name we derive the word hygiene. While Asclepius represents the masculine archetype of repairing the body, the goddess Hygieia personifies the feminine archetype of innate healing and prevention of disease.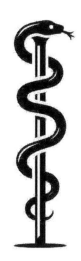

Holistic forms of Western medicine such as naturopathy retain both masculine and feminine aspects of healing, but conventional procedures and prescribing of drugs are tilted toward Asclepian medicine. Of course, one paradigm of medicine without the other does not allow us to thrive any more than a bird can fly with one wing. Integrative medicine requires that brain, body, and heart awareness work together to best heal the patient, the planet, and the relationship between the two.

With that in mind as well as our working definition that both cancer and trauma are wounds that aren't healing, we can begin the journey of answering why these wounds endure and how the path to healing trauma has a lot in common with healing from, and beyond, cancer.

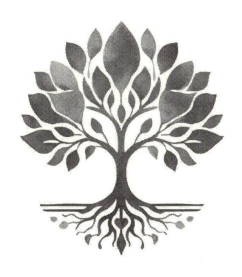

PART 1

The Cancer-Trauma Connection

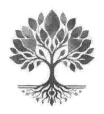

1

THE COMMON THREAD

"We have been wrong about what our job is in medicine. We think our job is to ensure health and survival. But really, it is larger than that. It is to enable well-being. And well-being is about the reasons one wishes to be alive."

—Atul Gawande, MD, from *Being Mortal*

That trauma and cancer share a common cause was not a foreign concept to the physicians of ancient Greece. Hippocrates, who is considered the father of Western medicine, introduced humoral theory. This theory posited that the human body has four fluids: blood, phlegm, yellow bile, and black bile. That imbalances in the humors cause illness is a quaint notion by modern biomedical standards, yet classical Grecian doctors were not wholly unscientific in their observations. A yellow-skinned jaundice patient was thought to be suffering from an excess of yellow bile—an apt diagnosis, even if the underlying cause was then unknown.

Thus, it should give us pause when the great Greek physician Claudius Galen upheld that the most virulent fluid, black bile, was the causative agent underlying two diseases: depression and cancer. "Indeed, *melancholia*, the medieval name for 'depression,' would draw its name from the Greek *melas*, 'black,' and *khole*, 'bile,'" writes Siddhartha Mukherjee, MD, in his opus *Cancer: The Emperor of All Maladies*.

While we associate depression with mental health and cancer with physical health, they believed that both have a common origin in pervasive toxicity. With environmental carcinogens causing aberrant gene mutations, this description of carcinogenesis is self-evident. That depression, anxiety, and trauma derive from a systemic psychological poison is less well appreciated.

Connecting the two disease states to a single causative agent is all the more compelling in light of another aspect of Greek medicine further elucidated by Mukherjee: "*Onkos* was the Greek term for a mass or a load, or more commonly a burden; cancer was imagined as a burden carried by the body."[1]

Galen was onto something. The line between physical, mental, and emotional is a blurry one, and while conventional medicine looks very different today than it did in ancient Greece, traditional medicine throughout Asia has retained an appreciation for the unity of being. It is more precise to state that the divide never existed in the first place—in either ancient Greece or

China—and it wasn't until much later that reductionist thinking suppressed the holistic paradigm of the ancient world.

When we state that a disease is "systemic," instead of thinking "throughout the body," we should consider it a disease process stemming from imbalances within the varied but unified expression of body, mind, and spirit.

Cancer and depression (and I would argue, most mental illnesses) are systemic. Though it may be possible to excise a malignant tumor, the underlying disease process known as cancer may go unchecked. As will become increasingly clear, cancer is often rooted in trauma, with the whole of one's being bearing the burden.

As we weave the common threads of cancer and trauma, it is helpful to differentiate stress from trauma and further define the prevalence of trauma in the postmodern world.

The effects of chronic stress can be beneficial or detrimental; it is akin to throwing pebbles into a pond. Ripples form but quickly dissipate, and it takes repeated events to effect a change. This is why exercise must be routine to have long-term benefits and why daily cigarette smoking accrues damage to lung tissue over the course of years.

Trauma is an emotional tsunami whereby the effects of a single incident can potentially be felt for the rest of one's life and can even be intergenerational in influence. It's dropping a boulder into a pond that displaces a portion of water. To heal, one must replenish the water that is the Heart-mind.

Not that chronic stress doesn't play a role in the cancer story and that the onus is all on traumatic experiences. As I detailed in my book *Cancer, Stress & Mindset*, chronic stress contributes to carcinogenesis by eroding resilience and promoting cancer growth.

"We know that chronic stress, whatever its source, puts the nervous system on edge, distorts the hormonal apparatus, impairs immunity, promotes inflammation, and undermines physical and mental well-being," writes Gabor Maté, MD, in his authoritative tome *The Myth of Normal: Trauma, Illness & Healing in a Toxic Culture*.

In some ways, the story of stress was easier for me to tell because we can readily measure the effects of chronic stress by testing cortisol levels or measuring heart rate variability. Healing trauma begins by learning how to cope with and mitigate the degrading influence of daily stresses. Leading from a more resilient state of being helps one face the challenges of past traumas, those episodes in life that undermine our ability to feel safe.

By that definition, few will make it into adulthood without multiple minor, if not major, traumatic events.

"Research by the Centers for Disease Control and Prevention has shown that one in five Americans was sexually molested as a child; one in four was beaten by a parent to the point of a mark being left on their body; and one in three couples engages in physical violence. A quarter of us grew up with alcoholic relatives, and one out of eight witnessed their mother being beaten or hit," reports psychiatrist Bessel van der Kolk, MD, in his seminal work on trauma, *The Body Keeps the Score: Brain, Mind, and Body in the Healing of Trauma.*

Traumatic experiences such as these have broad implications for mental health and create a susceptibility to addiction, but widespread trauma endemic to Western society also has devastating effects on the human immune system and sows the seeds for cancer.

That trauma can lead to chronic illness was previously relegated to the fringes of scientific research during the latter half of the 20th century and has only recently become widely acknowledged. Trauma research received mainstream recognition in a 2000 paper in the journal *Nature Neuroscience* that provided evidence that experiencing strong negative emotions, such as those elicited when recalling or reliving trauma, significantly changes parts of the brain that receive signals from viscera such as the gut, muscles, and skin.[2]

What is documented here is the connection—and therefore the possibility of disconnection—between body and brain with traumatic experience. This research invites us to consider that resolving trauma may require a somatic intervention, a therapy focused on integrating what the body is experiencing with what the brain is perceiving.

Posttraumatic Stress Disorder

A mature recognition of the body-mind connection took time to become established. Decades prior, the diverse symptoms associated with trauma were being recognized in the plight of Vietnam veterans. *Posttraumatic stress disorder (PTSD)* became a household term in the 1980s when New York-based psychoanalysts Chaim Shatan and Robert Lifton petitioned the American Psychiatric Association to include the diagnosis in the third edition of the *Diagnostic and Statistical Manual of Mental Dis-orders (DSM)*. With upwards of one quarter of veterans serving in war zones expected to develop PTSD, this was a problem screaming for societal acknowledgement.[3,4]

In modern parlance, PTSD connotes an experience that perpetuates feeling unsafe via conscious or subconscious triggers. Sometimes that trigger is obvious to the traumatized individual, such as a military veteran experiencing flashbacks to a foreign conflict when hearing the boom of fireworks.

The mainstream psychiatric diagnosis of PTSD as defined by the fifth edition of the DSM (*DSM-5*) includes eight required criteria of symptoms that have endured for longer than a month. A combat veteran being triggered by fireworks is called "intrusion." This refers to the sensory stimuli that launch a traumatized individual into sensations and feelings, similar to what occurred during the precipitating event. This can include flashbacks, nightmares, anxiety, or depression.

If anxiety, depression, or generalized agitation manifest with no obvious trigger, they are considered symptoms of hyperarousal. This manifestation of symptoms can be as debilitating as acute intrusive events because of their chronic nature. As resilience diminishes because of unresolved trauma, ongoing, low-level hyperarousal symptoms can rob one of a happy and meaningful life.

In a similar vein is the behavior of avoidance, a subset of symptoms that erodes the ability to have normal social interactions. Fear and shame alter behavior if they threaten to conjure memories of a past trauma, particularly if conditions feel similar to the circumstances surrounding the originating event. That may manifest as avoiding the intersection of an injurious motor vehicle accident, or refusing to drive on a dark and stormy night just like the one years ago when that crash occurred.

Another category of symptoms is a pervasive negativity that colors all future interactions. Consider physical or sexual abuse that degrades the victim's self-esteem and ability to have a healthy, intimate relationship. It can be a challenge to feel safe when an ongoing narrative of negativity overrides rational thinking. The higher brain is getting hijacked by an amygdala and hippocampus that insist survival is being threatened by entering a relationship. If those brain structures are unfamiliar, you'll learn more about how the brain processes trauma in a later section dedicated to neuroimaging.

It is important to point out that not everyone who endures a traumatic experience would describe the lingering effects as "stress" as denoted in the term posttraumatic stress disorder. At the level of the nervous system, some experience a hyperarousal of sympathetic activity and suffer from anxiety, while others will experience imbalanced dorsal vagal activity of the parasympathetic nervous system and struggle with depression.

In his book *Accessing the Healing Power of the Vagus Nerve: Self-Help Exercises for Anxiety, Depression, Trauma, and Autism*, manual therapist Stanley Rosenberg states that it "would be more accurate to talk about two different outcomes after a trauma: chronic, posttraumatic, spinal sympathetic activation state (the fight-or-flight stress response) or a posttraumatic state of chronic dorsal vagal activity (withdrawal or shut down)."[5]

I agree with this keen clinical insight by Rosenberg. An individual struggling with fear, apathy, helplessness, and depression should be treated differently than one with anxiety and flashback episodes. Instead, PTSD is the main trauma-related entry within the *DSM* that doesn't differentiate the two.

Another problem in recognizing and treating trauma is that the conditions that are more commonly diagnosed (and medicated for) are often the downstream consequences of trauma: anxiety, depression, and addiction. We think of these as separate and occasionally overlapping diagnosable conditions, but holistic medicine sees a deeper truth. These states are often branches extending from the same root of trauma.

A good question is why does a person experience anxiety and depression? A better question is what previous life experience have predisposed those states? A good question is why does a person have addiction? A better question is what emotional pain is the person self-medicating for? At the root of all these conditions and behaviors, it is not uncommon to find trauma.

At face value, the diagnosis of PTSD acknowledges a trauma has occurred and that symptoms persist because of it, but instead of treating people by their common trauma, we group them by their maladaptive behavior or symptom presentation. Thus we have support groups for various addictions, such as eating disorders or alcoholism, even if the trauma that drove those individuals to binge eat or abuse alcohol may be vastly different.

It would make more sense to identify the trauma, such as childhood neglect or verbal abuse, and allow patients to heal (as groups or privately) in connection with those adverse formative experiences. In this way, the cause can be addressed as readily as the downstream effect.

This doesn't mean that certain chemical addictions won't require medical intervention for the symptoms of withdrawal—they certainly will and must—but ancillary to that would be honoring the person's history and space to address the underlying and predisposing traumas. This does not differ from a cancer patient in active treatment. Medical intervention is necessary, but a broader holistic approach to healing would invite that cancer patient to uncover the emotional and spiritual roots of disease and dysfunction.

Here's one example for now, with more to follow: A 2019 study in *Cancer Research* showed that women with PTSD were twice as likely to be diagnosed with ovarian cancer, even 26 years later (the prospective duration of the study). Looking over the data, the more severe the trauma history, quantified by number and duration of PTSD symptoms, the stronger the association with more aggressive cancer types.[6]

Another problem with relying solely on textbook criteria that define PTSD is that not everyone with a trauma history develops PTSD, but this doesn't make that adverse experience any less potent. Sometimes a patient's story doesn't check every box for PTSD according to the *DSM*, but the effects of trauma may still be omnipresent and subtly undermining one's sense of self and safety, even if not overtly debilitating.

Nor does the *DSM* contain a means to evaluate societal trauma. With acts of war or terrorism, we may be quick to triage the most severe physical and psychological damage without an appreciation for the suffering of those tangentially connected to the event. This is not unlike the emotional suffering experienced by caregivers after a close friend or family member receives a dire cancer diagnosis. We're quick to tend to the needs of the cancer patient, while a dearth of support exists for the caregiver.

After almost 20 years in clinical practice, I've learned that a diagnosis is only as useful as the awareness it creates and the treatment options it empowers. Describing a problem is not enough. The very act of diagnosing needs to be an act of healing—or at least the first step in a healing journey.

LIVING WITH SMALL BOWEL OBSTRUCTIONS

I remember when I first realized that I had PTSD. While a psychotherapist might disregard my self-diagnosis, I don't think it's any more complicated than realizing a past trauma is altering one's present ability to function normally.

In my case, I was sprawled out on the bathroom floor having an episode of a small bowel obstruction (SBO). The intense twisting abdominal pain, nausea, and vomiting lasted throughout the night, and I was physically and emotionally drained when I could again be coherent. This was a scene that played out several times before the trip to the emergency room that resulted in my lymphoma diagnosis.

In those first few years after remission, these episodes continued to occur, each time triggering the same terrifying implication by association—an SBO episode meant abdominal tumors had returned. After several clear CT scans, I was left with the fortunate/unfortunate realization that such episodes were being caused by adhesions, scar tissue that persisted despite the resolution of the tumors.

It was a relief to confirm that an SBO episode did not equate to a cancer relapse, yet I still had the reminder of all the uncertainty, physical pain, and emotional destabili-zation that followed such an episode. That's when I realized how PTSD was manifesting in my life, though the word "stress" in "post-traumatic stress disorder" is not strong enough language.

For every veteran that cringes at the sound of fireworks, for every domestic violence victim that cowers upon hearing a raised voice, and for every cancer patient that is shaking while slowly shuffling to the chemotherapy room, "stress" does not describe the intensity of the moment.

What I experienced on the bathroom floor and what every traumatized human experiences when triggered is a "retraumatization." A better acronym would be "PTT" for "posttraumatic trauma."

The point is that trauma can perpetuate itself in predictable and unpredictable ways. There are elements of a trauma history that are overt provocations, and then there are the moments of being blindsided by a new trigger. Low levels of stress and anxiety may accompany an individual in the months and years following a traumatic event, but there are also debilitating memories and feelings that hijack the ability to think clearly and rationally. There is more to the human journey than can be encapsulated by the term "PTSD."

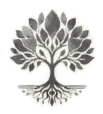

2

THE SHOCK TO THE SYSTEM

"Trauma is what happens inside of you because of what happens to you. It is the internal response to the external event."

—Gabor Maté, MD

Presently, *DSM-5* defines trauma as: "Exposure to actual or threatened death, serious injury, or sexual violence in one (or more) of the following ways: directly experiencing the traumatic event(s); witnessing, in person, the traumatic event(s) as it occurred to others; learning that the traumatic event(s) occurred to a close family member or close friend (in case of actual or threatened death of a family member or friend, the event(s) must have been violent or accidental); or experiencing repeated or extreme exposure to aversive details of the traumatic event(s)."

The emphasis of this definition is on the physical, yet there are many situations that don't involve enduring or witnessing a physical threat but are emotionally destabilizing. Repeated verbal abuse is one such example; neglect is another.

Then there is the history of the individual experiencing the traumatic event.

"I will maintain that the implied threat is based more on its meaning to the individual based on prior traumatic experiences than its intrinsic severity," writes neurologist and trauma researcher Robert Scaer, MD, in his book *The Body Bears the Burden*.

Scaer is among many traumatologists who have suggested that dissociation, not physical injury, is the defining characteristic of trauma. Dissociation is a shock to the system that overwhelms our ability to respond. With a threat, the sympathetic nervous system is engaged, preparing the individual to fight or flee. When overwhelmed, animals of many species, including humans, will freeze and feign death. This is a survival response initiated by the parasympathetic nervous system.

A freeze response can produce such a profound state of dissociation that the victim may not even feel the physical pain associated with trauma as the body is flooded with endorphins. Contrast this with the high-adrenaline sympathetic activation that feeds the fight-or-flight response.[1]

"Dissociation at the time of a traumatic experience predicts the later development of PTSD more than any other measured variable," according to van der Kolk.[2]

A freeze response leading to dissociation describes a mental state characterized by a disruption of conscious awareness, including such experiences as altered perception of time and space, lapses in memory, and loss of identity. In the most extreme form, this results in dissociative identity disorder, whereby distinct personalities emerge from the same consciousness.

In other instances, the moment of trauma can give rise to an out-of-body experience as consciousness dissociates. This raises the question of what consciousness is and how loosely it is tethered to the body. We'll explore the implications of such phenomena later.

What is most relevant to a mature understanding of PTSD is the context in which it occurs. If the victim is a child who experiences a profound shock to the system, the resultant dissociation may arrest developmental maturity. That emotional development can be hampered is itself a defining characteristic of dissociation. Why this happens is as much a feature of the helplessness of the individual as the severity of the threat. The combination is key to triggering dissociation, and children, being the most vulnerable, are much more likely to feel helpless with threats that adults could more easily manage. But that loss of autonomy in the child is a theme that may reverberate throughout their life and set the stage for future physical and mental illness.

Another feature of dissociation is the repression of traumatic memories, as is often the case with sexual trauma. Painful memories may then resurface years later with a triggering event that causes details of the original trauma to flood back into conscious awareness.[3]

How accurate those memories are is beside the point. The relived experience of them is very real. Unfortunately, recalling a traumatic experience doesn't magically resolve it. Awareness opens the door to healing, but talk therapy around the traumatic narrative doesn't ensure that flashbacks and the related visceral symptoms will subside.

"If the problem with PTSD is dissociation, the goal of treatment would be association: integrating the cut-off elements of the trauma into the ongoing narrative of life," is the wise counsel of van der Kolk.[4]

Developmental Trauma

Developmental trauma illustrates why talk therapy is sometimes insufficient for trauma resolution. A preverbal child stores trauma subconsciously, or even unconsciously, in procedural memory. This is a body-based, or somatic, long-term memory expressed in feelings rather than thoughts or words. Contrast this with a trauma experienced by an older child or adult. The ability to build a narrative around the event grounds the incident in declarative memory, where new thoughts can further shape one's perception of the trauma. This is simply not possible with a developmental trauma experienced by a preverbal child or infant. Accessing and healing from it must occur at a visceral level.

Developmental trauma can begin in utero with maternal

stress. Authors Robin Karr-Morse and Meredith S. Wiley cover this topic in detail in their exemplary book *Scared Sick: The Role of Childhood Trauma in Adult Disease*. Referencing animal research and human observational studies, they offer: "Maternal stress during pregnancy is highly correlated with spontaneous abortion, pre-eclampsia, preterm birth, low birth weight and the adult diseases that follow these conditions."

This will sound as bizarre as it barbaric, but it took until the late 80s to determine that infants could feel pain. Before that, the conventional belief was that a lack of developmental nerve myelination precluded the sensory experience of pain, or at least the memory of it.

Thus, until about 1986, babies receiving cardiac surgery were only put in temporary paralysis but not given anesthesia. Imagine how the helplessness experienced during an excruciatingly painful surgery lasting multiple hours imprints on the psyche of an infant. Although neonatal cardiac surgery is a rare event—and is now performed under anesthesia—consider the far more common event in newborn boys of circumcision in which genital mutilation was typically practiced without anesthesia until 1999. The doctor immobilized the baby and clamped the foreskin before quickly excising it with a scalpel.

As a child ages, the most likely source of trauma is parental abuse and neglect, an insidious and underappreciated source of lifelong mental and physical health struggles. This can take many forms and carries through into adulthood.

Physical abuse is violence perpetrated against an individual by threat, action, or both. The pain endured is as much emotional as physical. Verbal abuse and debasement result in deep emotional scarring, particularly when experienced over an extended time. The chronic nature of verbal abuse can be just as devastating to an impressionable child as physical abuse. Sexual abuse is an awful combination of physical and emotional trauma that violates every aspect of personal safety and well-being and almost assuredly results in dissociation at any age. Finally, if a religious leader commits sexual abuse, it also inflicts spiritual abuse by eroding the victim's sense of purity and holiness.

Abuse can also occur through neglect. Absence of care can be as damaging as attention given through verbal or physical abuse.

"Over the years our research team has repeatedly found that chronic emotional abuse and neglect can be just as devastating as physical abuse and sexual molestation," van der Kolk stated.[5]

Sadly, some children grow up in an environment alternating between the two: neglect for long stretches escalating to moments of intense physical, verbal, and/or sexual abuse. Of the 3 million US children reported as victims of neglect or abuse, a third of them require the intervention of child protective services. That's 1 million children, annually, experiencing the trauma of endangerment in their own homes.[6]

Developmental trauma has the added concern of affecting the brain while it is most receptive and vulnerable. This explains, in part, why negative experiences during childhood can have lasting implications on mental stability and physical resilience into adulthood. This line of thinking underlies the connection between childhood trauma and chronic disease in adults.

To understand how this might occur, one area of research focuses on changes in the brain that become deeply entrenched when trauma is experienced at an impressionable young age. Martin Teicher, MD, PhD, studied this very subject as director of the Developmental Biopsychiatry Research Program at McLean Hospital in Belmont, Massachusetts.

Stress and trauma are processed by the limbic system of the brain, particularly the amygdala. This region can become dys-regulated under the influence of chronic elevated levels of the stress hormone cortisol, but that effect is magnified by the dis-sociative effect of trauma. Moreover, if that trauma occurs during a critical period in early development, the neurocircuitry of PTSD can persist into adulthood.[7,8]

Developmental trauma presents additional hurdles to over-come, given the unconscious processing of the triggering event and its long-term storage in procedural memory. The contrast to this is declarative memory. These are the two sides of the coin that is long-term memory.

Procedural memory is unconscious and somatic, tied heavily to the function of the autonomic nervous system. This explains how a past trauma can unknowingly elicit symptoms (increased heart rate, shallow breathing), even without knowledge of the trig-ger. Panic attacks can be like that for some people. One moment someone is going about his or her merry way, and then some external trigger blindsides the person, escalating anxiety.

Other times the trigger can be much more subtle, such as hearing a song that was played during a close friend's funeral years ago. You may have long forgotten the connection, but suddenly grief surfaces as the subconscious relives the feelings tied to that event.

While procedural memory is implicit, declarative memory is explicit. Declarative memory involves remembering factual information that can be described in a cohesive narrative, often using language. If traumatic memories were only stored in declarative memory, talk therapy would be sufficient to rewrite the narrative of the painful event and create a healing relationship to it.

Clinical researchers made an interesting discovery that sheds light on why we must address developmental trauma differently by studying the integration between the two hemispheres of the brain in adults with and without a history of childhood trauma. When recalling either a neutral or disturbing memory, adults without a history of trauma displayed activity in both sides of the brain. By contrast, subjects with a history of developmental trauma showed dominant left-hemisphere processing with neutral memories and right-hemisphere dominance with disturbing memories.[9]

This suggests an inherent brain imbalance called laterality. Those with a history of PTSD have an atrophied corpus callosum, which magnifies the effect because it is the aspect of brain anatomy that connects the hemispheres of the brain.[10]

These collective findings point to a fundamental breakdown

in how the brain processes developmental trauma. This explains how procedural memory experiences and stores trauma in the body-mind and why therapists have introduced different forms of therapy to bridge the gap between the somatic (or visceral) experience of trauma and our ability to rationalize it. We'll learn more about this in the therapies section.

It is important to emphasize that trauma stored in procedural memory is not restricted to preverbal developmental experiences. Adults with the full capacity to think, speak, and rationalize cannot process trauma if the event is severe enough to cause dissociation. By definition, dissociation denotes an inability to have a conscious grasp of a traumatic experience. The conscious mind checks out as a survival mechanism, while the body takes the brunt of the trauma.

It should now be patently obvious that dissociation and developmental trauma are massive deterrents to optimal health and well-being, but the trauma-cancer connection becomes even more apparent when adding epigenetics into the mix.

Intergenerational Trauma

"The fathers have eaten sour grapes, and the children's teeth are set on edge."

—Ezekiel 18:2

Can trauma be passed on to subsequent generations? Answering that question has become the research focus of Rachel Yehuda, PhD, a professor of psychiatry and neuroscience and director of the Traumatic Stress Studies Division at Mount Sinai School of Medicine. Her work on the science of epigenetics gets to the heart of trauma and its connection to cancer.

Developmental biologist Conrad Waddington coined the term "epigenetics." It literally means "above the genome" and describes the means by which genes turn on or off from external factors. Both developmental and environmental triggers can alter gene expression, so an appreciation of this process is necessary to understand how trauma can shape biology.

Environmental factors influence the expression of genes, indicating the human genome is not fixed. It is the "nurture" to the "nature" we are born with, suggesting that some disease states, like cancer, will become more or less likely given certain external pressures. This is true of exposure to carcinogens turning on oncogenes and turning off tumor-suppressing genes but is also true of trauma affecting the expression of genes.

Only 5–10% of cancers are caused by an inherited genetic defect, meaning that at least 90% of all cancers are epigenetic in origin. Simply put, cancer isn't a genetically deterministic disease.[11]

The conventional thinking used to be (and still is in some circles) that random mutations give rise to a precancerous cell. Left unchecked by the immune system, a nest of rogue cells grows into a tumor. If the cause of mutations were truly random, then we could speak in terms of luck regarding who develops cancer and who does not. Perhaps these mishaps of genetics will occur in anyone who lives long enough as an effect of the aging process?

Yet the science of epigenetics points to the fact that anything that challenges the body through oxidative stress or direct damage to DNA has the potential to kick-start the formation of tumors. Genetic predispositions may explain susceptibilities to certain kinds of cancer, but the expression of those genes is caused by environmental triggers in the majority of cases. Genes load the gun, but environment pulls the trigger.

Now consider the possibility that epigenetic effects can be passed on to future generations. As early as 1999, biologist Emma Whitelaw demonstrated that epigenetic marks could be passed from one generation of mice to the next. Her seminal work with mice challenged the notion that epigenetic effects are cleared from access to the germ line in mammals, and thus only genetic traits could be inherited.[12]

The same principle appears to be true with traumatic events, where Yehuda's research suggests that the effects of trauma may cause epigenetic changes sufficient to alter gene expression in future generations. This notion was documented in a 2016 paper studying the intergenerational effects of methylation of a specific gene in Holocaust survivors. This was followed up by a larger study in 2020 that replicated the findings.[13,14]

Additional research with Holocaust survivors elucidates the breadth of these epigenetic changes, with dozens of genes found to be significantly affected. These epigenetic changes predominantly result in a downregulation of immune function and increased activity of—and sensitivity to, cortisol, the adrenal glands' primary hormone for mitigating long-term stress.[15] These are significant biochemical markers for physiological shifts that promote cancer growth.[16]

The gist of these findings is that trauma changes the body as much as it does the mind and emotions, and the science of epigenetics explains how that might be happening. Even more compelling is research with expectant mothers who experienced significant trauma. Yehuda examined the effects of PTSD on pregnant women who survived the terrorist attacks on the World Trade Center.[17]

When measuring salivary cortisol levels in mother and child nine months postpartum, her findings suggest that pregnant women who developed PTSD in response to the attacks had lower cortisol levels, as did their babies. The effect was most noticeable in babies born to mothers who suffered trauma during their third trimester. This stands in contrast to the control group of pregnant women who experienced the attacks but did not develop PTSD and had normal cortisol output.

Trauma has a paradoxical effect on stress resilience; developmental trauma sometimes predisposes the child to either elevated or depressed levels of cortisol through adulthood. It is unclear why, but may have to do with the timing of the trauma, whether fetal or within the first few years of life, and other genetic predispositions.[18]

Transference is not limited to mothers. Micro-RNA are ribonucleic acid (RNA) fragments that bind to messenger RNA and alter protein synthesis. Research has shown that micro-RNA found in the sperm of male mice can both convey traumatic experience and modify gene expression in their offspring, with analogous effects studied in human men.[19]

It is well established that trauma affects future generations, and this is a result of both nature and nurture. Consider someone struggling with the debilitating symptoms of PTSD from being raised by a traumatized parent. Left untreated, PTSD perpetuates cycles of violence and abuse as trauma begets trauma.[20]

The question remains: Is this effect a learned behavior, or is the epigenetic shift that Yehuda's team is observing truly inherited? Animal research suggests the latter may be the case.

When mice were traumatized to the point of erratic behavior, the researchers observed that their offspring exhibited similar behavior, according to a 2010 paper by University of Zurich professor of neuroepigenetics Isabelle Mansuy, PhD.[21]

Of course, this is not sufficient evidence to tease apart the nature vs. nurture components of the erratic behavior; the next generation of mice could have inherited the trait by observation. Researchers then controlled for this effect by breeding traumatized male mice with untraumatized females and let the offspring mature without interaction with the males. Stunningly, the pups of the traumatized male mice exhibited abnormal behavior.[22]

Just three years later, researchers performed a remarkably

clever experiment that further strengthens the argument that traumatic memory can be passed down epigenetically. Researchers "fear conditioned" mice to a specific odor and then noted that the two subsequent generations also negatively responded to the same odor, even in the absence of the traumatic conditioning.[23]

If this effect is true for humans, it would imply that one's grandchildren can inherit an aversion associated with a traumatic experience. There is some indication in the research literature that this effect is not limited to mice and that infants exposed to stressful situations or neglect can pass on epigenetic changes to their children.[24]

Collectively, these findings build a strong case that human trauma can be inherited on an epigenetic level. Combine this with the cycles of abuse that get passed on as behaviors, and a picture emerges where multiple influences shape the transmission of trauma to future generations.

The term transgenerational implies the nature and nurture totality of epigenetic transference on offspring, both good and bad. And that's the good news: Healing can be passed on just as surely as trauma. We'll explore the research—and hope—of healing the transgressions of the past in the strategies section.

3

THE BIOPSYCHOSOCIAL MODEL

"Imagine the feeling of relief that would flood our whole being if we knew that when we were in the grip of sorrow or illness, our village would respond to our need. This would not be out of pity, but out of a realization that every one of us will take our turn at being ill, and we will need one another. The indigenous thought is when one of us is ill, all of us are ill."

—Francis Weller from *The Wild Edge of Sorrow*

Society burdens us, perpetuating trauma in many instances, but healthy relationships are a powerful avenue of healing. The biopsychosocial model is a holistic approach to wellness introduced by psychiatrist George Engel, MD, in the 1970s. To an understanding of human physiology, it adds the impact of relationships, both with oneself and others, as a driving cause and cure of disease.

We give credence to "social ills" with little appreciation for how they create individual illness. Consider the crippling impact of loneliness. A 2010 meta-analysis examining the pooled risk factors of over 300,000 participants found that strong social support was a better predictor of survival than other lifestyle factors we are typically concerned about: smoking, alcohol consumption, blood pressure, and body mass index.[1]

If this study is worth its salt, it would speak to the massive elephant in the room for many people: Loneliness is a cause of disease, and social support is the cure.[2]

This truth is self-evident from personal experience. I recall being diagnosed with cancer and quickly realizing that it would take support from my extended family and local community if I were to stay positive considering the dire circumstances I was facing.

So, too, it is with a history of trauma that society has perpetrated, whether by the words and actions of a random stranger or by someone in our home. Trauma rarely occurs in an isolated bubble. The wound that isn't healing—the wound of cancer and trauma—invites us to see the bigger picture of wholeness within society, demanding a biopsychosocial model of healing.

With that in mind, it is worthwhile to zoom out and layer human evolution onto the biopsychosocial model of trauma. A 2003 paper by Michael Christopher, PhD, titled "A Broader View of Trauma: A Biopsychosocial-Evolutionary View of the Role of the Traumatic Stress Response in the Emergence of Pathology and/or Growth" adds a critical concept to this discussion.

Christopher wisely acknowledges that trauma, ubiquitous to life, is best understood as an evolutionary inherited mechanism for growth, enabling adaptation and proper development. When we view stress, anxiety, and trauma through this lens, we can transform them into learning. Healthy social relationships reinforce this learning.

Lawrence G. Calhoun and Richard G. Tedeschi introduced the notion of an adaptive response to trauma, called posttraumatic growth (PTG), in the 1990s. Christopher adds this concept into a larger biopsychosocial-evolutionary context because it highlights certain clinical implications. The most obvious is that trauma is essential to our ability to adapt as a species. In other words, you can't separate human suffering from human achievement. How we manage and collectively heal from trauma determines the extent of our cultural enlightenment.

Christopher also astutely points out that, while "pharmacological treatment may be helpful in lowering traumatic stress by modulating the HPA axis, it may also interfere with the normal process of neural pruning and reconfiguration that is essential to PTG. Therefore, if the clinical goal of trauma treatment is to facilitate PTG rather than simply minimizing symptoms, as this perspective suggests it should be, pharmacological intervention should be used very sparingly in the case of trauma exposure."[3]

What, then, are the impediments to PTG within a broader biopsychosocial-evolutionary context?

Shame and Guilt

Seeing trauma as a shared human experience is the first step. Recognizing the deterrents to engaging with supportive, healing relationships is the next.

There is an emotional backdrop that perpetuates the suppression of traumatic memories precluding biopsychosocial healing of trauma. What exactly are these emotions that impede the acknowledgement and assimilation of trauma?

In two words: shame and guilt.

There is a subtle difference in how shame and guilt are defined. Both share the experience of feeling blame, but guilt reflects someone's internal experience, while shame is a projection on to the individual. They often go together, as public shaming of an individual causes them to feel and perpetuate guilt, ultimately stunting emotional expression.

Some cultures use shame as a form of cultural currency. I experienced this firsthand during my travels in Asia. To deviate too far from the norm or dishonor one's family can elicit public shaming in many Asian cultures. By contrast, I reflect upon my Italian Catholic heritage that (seemingly) values guilt as a necessary ingredient in cultivating saintly behavior.

Consider both concepts in the context of a sexual trauma. A woman who is the victim of rape may struggle with projections of shame if she received messages that the way she acted or dressed brought the incident on. She may then internalize this messaging and consider the rape partially her fault. To be clear with this example: In no way does a woman's behavior ever justify a man's violation of her body. Yet these feelings of guilt and shame can feed denial of trauma within the fabric of society and within the psyche of a rape victim.

The salient point here is that trauma can shatter what it means to feel safe. With that comes a maligning of emotional expression—perpetuating shame and guilt, living in fear, inappropriate outbursts of anger—and this in turn colors our decisions, including the impulse to seek help.

If we are to overcome trauma as individuals and heal as a society, we have to first own the fact that we all hurt one another. Sometimes that hurt is intentional, and often it is not, but trauma begets more trauma because we are all individuals struggling to heal amidst adversity.

For a committed individual, a supportive care team can help heal deep emotional wounding without the involvement of close family and friends. However, that healing can extend into family constellations and communities if we acknowledge the hurt within ourselves and how our actions may have hurt others. It takes a village, and as each weak link in the chain of our community heals, so does the integrity of the web of our interconnectedness.

This is a critical factor for a newly diagnosed cancer patient. The detrimental trend that can arise from shame and guilt surrounding cancer treatment is to decline community support or even decide not to tell extended family, friends, and coworkers of the diagnosis.

If undergoing rigorous conventional oncology treatment, it would be hard to hide the fact that one is a cancer patient, but I have seen patients who undergo therapies with less obvious side effects choose to not disclose their diagnosis. They may even pass off a week's absence from work for a surgical lumpectomy as a planned vacation.

I respect that an introverted cancer patient will need plenty of alone time to reflect. This is certainly still true for even the more extroverted among us, but asking for privacy when community support can respond to many small needs is cutting off a significant opportunity for healing.

For those who open themselves to help, a meal drop-off or offer to clean the house can be a boon. I needed to take some time off from the clinic when I was first diagnosed and didn't hesitate to explain the situation to my patients. The get-well cards I received from friends, family, and patients were heartening, and I still have them hanging up in my office to remind me of all the prayers of support that helped carry me through those difficult first several months.

Feeling shame about being sick may underlie the choice to decline help. Having to bow out of one's responsibilities can dishearten someone whose identity is wrapped up in being strong and reliable. This is most evident in moms juggling caregiving for young children while now suddenly needing lots of care themselves. It is also true of an independent elderly person now requiring help for the first time in their adult life. Nobody wants to be a burden, but a cancer journey is one best not walked alone.

Trauma victims and cancer patients alike can also exhibit the "poor-me" syndrome as the flip side of this.

Victim Consciousness

When a person is overwhelmed by trauma, they may believe that the world is unsafe. This is especially true of a cancer patient in remission, fearful of relapse.

A victim mindset has broad implications, with two common manifestations. The first took center stage with author Caroline Myss in her book *Anatomy of the Spirit: The Seven Stages of Power and Healing.* Myss purports that traumatized individuals may identify with their physical, emotional, or psychological wounds and use them to gain sympathy, avoid responsibility, or maintain a sense of control in their lives. When we treat our history as a form of cultural currency, it prevents us from realizing genuine, lasting healing.

Take, for example, a cancer patient who declines an invitation to a social event by proclaiming that, because of having a cancer history, they'd rather avoid large groups of people and risk getting sick. That might be an accurate sentiment, but what they were really thinking is "I'd rather stay home and take a bath." Instead of leading with a strong statement of self-care, they leverage sympathy around their cancer history to hedge and avoid any challenge to their claim. The problem with this behavior is that it perpetuates the undercurrent of feeling unsafe with a self-fulfilling prophecy.

Sometimes the expression of victimization is subconscious.

Physician Bernie S. Siegel pioneered a therapy group called Exceptional Cancer Patients (ECaP) to help oncology patients live better and longer. In his book *Love, Medicine and Miracles*, Siegel offers that "Women whose children die young or who have unhappy love relationships are especially vulnerable to breast and cervical diseases. One ECaP patient, who had lost two husbands to cancer, had uterine cancer and herpes zoster (shingles) in one of her breasts. I don't think it was coincidence that, after two such losses, she developed diseases of two sex organs that would effectively keep other men away."[4]

The second manifestation of a victim mindset is less overt and more insidious. Trauma specialist Paul Conti, MD, speaks of "selective abstraction" as the tendency to have a great day spiral into negativity due to one unfortunate event. This underlies the shift in one's perception from positive with maybe a tinge of negativity to a complete rewrite of the day's narrative as awful because of one unfortunate circumstance at the tail end of the day.

Selective abstraction is more than garden-variety pessimism.

This is someone whose outlook is radically altered because trauma has rewired the ability to weave a fabric of positive when presented with one thread of negative. Perhaps you know someone like this; perhaps this describes you. This is a flavor of victim consciousness that hijacks our perception of goodness. Conti describes it as trauma's "master stroke—convincing us that it's our destiny to be on the receiving end of more trauma."

To be fair, it's hard to know when trauma is leading and when sympathy-seeking victim consciousness is running the show. Sometimes it's a bit of both. The difference is that victim consciousness plays out in the avoidance or recollection of positive experiences, while trauma revolves around the avoidance of and preoccupation with negative encounters.

Nipping victim consciousness in the bud takes brutal honesty and a commitment to thinking, speaking, and acting with integrity. If you need help to heal from cancer, ask for help. If you need time to rest, it's okay to bow out of all commitments. Even if most decisions are made for the sake of healing from cancer, that doesn't mean you have to explicitly make life about cancer. Make it about you. Make it about leaning into that which is positive rather than perpetuating negative circumstances.

This speaks to the ultimate antidote for victim consciousness: self-love. I will be the first to admit that loving oneself is difficult. The light of our personal truth can become shrouded by doubt and self-loathing. Many struggle with feeling worthy of love, mired in guilt from past wrongdoing. For some, this can be a seemingly insurmountable mountain of negative emotion to overcome.

If love seems unreachable, try compassion. When I reflect on the feeling of love, I think about a pet dog that responds to its people with complete loyalty and absence of judgment. Humans are seldom capable of that level of unconditional love.

Compassion is the ability to express care despite differences. It may be rooted in the empathy of shared struggle but could also be an expression of sympathy. Compassion offers the perspective that life is fraught with challenges endemic to the human codition. I can't understand the plight of a rabbit caught in a snare, but I can have compassion for the pain of struggling to escape a less-than-desirable situation.

Mentally stepping outside of oneself, it becomes easier to have compassion for our own struggles as we do for those of others. It's a subtle consciousness shift but carries with it a neutrality that makes it far easier to experience than unconditional love. Even if you can't see beyond the negative emotions that prevent access to unconditional love (of oneself or others), you can change the narrative of your inner dialogue and practice compassion.

It's not easy to forgive someone who hurt you, but it is easier to extend compassion when considering the probable trauma in the wrong doer's past. This doesn't mean society shouldn't convict perpetrators of egregious acts of harm, but opens the possibility to consider the history of the perpetrator that frees the victim from experiencing prolonged hatred. Even when forgiveness seems out of reach, having compassion for oneself means that the psychological impact of trauma does not continue to poison your thoughts and emotions.

Life is hard. We are hurt, and we hurt others. Few attain the idyllic state of sainthood, loving and forgiving unconditionally, but we are all capable of compassion. Don't let victim consciousness rob you of that peace; healing is just on the other side of compassion.

Distraction

"We labour at our daily work more ardently and thoughtlessly than is necessary to sustain our life because it is even more necessary not to have leisure to stop and think. Haste is universal because everyone is in flight from himself."

—Friedrich Nietzsche

Severe trauma is hard to forget, but even with our best efforts to do so, trauma gets suppressed only to emerge like a whale periodically surfacing for air. We think all is going swimmingly until a cascade of memories comes spouting out our emotional blowhole. If not prepared to deal with the deluge, distraction is an understandable coping mechanism.

What is less appreciated is how numbing distraction can be,

sometimes thwarting the full resolution of long-standing trauma. Consider the story of writer and self-proclaimed internet addict Andrew Sullivan. In his article in *New York* magazine titled "I Used to Be a Human Being," Sullivan describes his bittersweet love affair with social media and blogging several times a day. With a six-figure follower count, the drive to scour the internet and multitask himself to exhaustion led Sullivan to seek a meditation retreat for an extended digital detox.

All was initially going well after relinquishing his cellphone and walking or sitting for several hours a day in silent meditation. He describes feeling his body more intimately and listening to the sounds of nature instead of filtering out the background soundscape. Then something inexplicable happened for which he was not prepared. Memories surfaced of childhood trauma living with and without a mother with bipolar disorder. He recalled walking the halls of psychiatric institutions and her emotional breakdowns in his arms. These memories arose during a quiet walk in the woods that reminded Sullivan of where he grew up. His reflections are as universal as they are deeply personal:

> I knew the scar tissue from this formative trauma was still in my soul. I had spent two decades in therapy, untangling and exploring it, learning how it had made intimacy with others so frightening, how it had made my own spasms of adolescent depression even more acute, how living with that kind of pain from the most powerful source of love in my life had made me

the profoundly broken vessel I am. But I had never felt it so vividly since the very years it had first engulfed and defined me. It was as if, having slowly and progressively removed every distraction from my life, I was suddenly faced with what I had been distracting myself from. Resting for a moment against the trunk of a tree, I stopped, and suddenly found myself bent over, convulsed with the newly present pain, sobbing.

Counseling from a facilitator at the meditation retreat assured Sullivan that this catharsis was normal and would resolve with time. It did, with a softening that can occur in the fullness of time if one is not given a chance to suppress those difficult feelings with distractions.

This key insight from Sullivan's story is all too common in our hyperdistracted society and is a theme that keeps coming up in relation to trauma. Addictions can result from trauma but can also be an impediment to resolution. We initially adopt various addictions and distractions to blunt the pain of trauma and perpetuate them in a way that prevents access to those long-suppressed feelings.

Sullivan was in a safe place for his catharsis to surface, and even if he was unprepared for the manner and intensity in which traumatic memories arose, it occurred on his terms. This is a far better scenario than going about one's life—replete with distractions— and having an unforeseen triggering event open a traumatic wound. A cellphone dies or the box of cigarettes is empty, and being cut off while driving to the store to remedy the situation spirals into road rage. Is it any wonder how trauma perpetrates and perpetuates trauma?

It takes a lot of courage to acknowledge that we are all numbing ourselves against some chronic stress or deep-seated trauma. Facing discomfort after removing distractions requires even more courage.

The unflinching approach of a silent meditation retreat is not for everyone; it can be too painful to remove all distractions and rip off the bandage covering our deepest wounds. There is the option to experiment with longer and longer periods refraining from known distractions. That could take the form of a digital-detox day or weekend. It could be an extended fast from social media.

As Sullivan points out in the clever title of his article, many, if not all of us in the modern world used to be human beings. The ability to be connected, virtually, at all moments of our waking life has been the defining transition from being "human beings" to "human doings."

Trauma knocks softly; other times, it breaks the door down. How prepared we are to face what comes through the door depends a lot on whether we are alert and looking up or are staring, head down, into a screen of eternal distraction.

Even though Sullivan achieved these realizations in a contemplative environment without distractions, it is important to point out that he did not do so alone. The guidance within the meditation retreat enabled him to ground his insights within a larger social context. This is the promise of the biopsychosocial model of healing trauma.

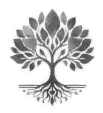

4

CONNECTING THE DOTS

"Traumatic stress is an illness of not being able to be fully alive in the present."

—Pierre Janet, 1889

The brain's response to stress and trauma highlights how easily it can become triggered by future events. Say you are walking down a suburban street at night and hear a rustle in a bush nearby. The likely response is to startle away from the bush given the unknown threat. Moments later, a feral cat hightails it out of the bush and streaks across the street. In the absence of harm, feelings of safety return. Meanwhile, you may still need to come down from the acute activation of the sympathetic nervous system. It may take a few moments for a rapid heart rate to return to normal and shallow breathing to deepen.

When the sensory organs of the body receive a powerful stimulus, the thalamus of the limbic system quickly signals the adjacent amygdala and the higher brain centers of the neocortex. The limbic system is the first responder, assessing threat before the thinking aspects of the neocortex have time to weigh in.

The amygdala triggers all the physiological changes necessary to prepare to encounter a challenge to survival. Norepinephrine (adrenaline) surges, and the body reacts before the neocortex can make a judgment based upon experience.

Neuroscientist Joseph LeDoux, PhD, calls this near instantaneous response by the limbic system the "low-road" response to a threat, and it responds faster than the "high-road" input of the rationalizing neocortex.[*]

Several other brain regions share the task of keeping us safe from a potential threat. The hippocampus is a part of the limbic system involved with memory that quickly compares a perceived threat against similar experiences. If a history of being bitten by a dog causes an involuntary jump at the sound of a nearby aggressive-sounding bark, the hippocampus contributed to that knee-jerk reaction.

The low-road limbic system response is universal and more common in those with a history of trauma. What makes PTSD so debilitating is how quickly anxiety can emerge from a multitude

---

[*] Researchers have varying estimates of how much faster the limbic system responds than the prefrontal cortex, depending on whether threat response is measured via functional magnetic resonance imaging (fMRI) or electroencephalogram (EEG).

of triggers. The loud bang of fireworks may cause a slight reaction in most but produce a dramatic flashback for a military veteran who experienced munitions conflict.

With unresolved trauma, that reaction is immediate, physiological, and seemingly beyond conscious control. It feels that way because the brain is preparing the body long before the rational brain gets a handle of the situation. If the trigger is sufficient to throw the person into a full-fledged episode of fear and anxiety, the rational higher brain may never get a chance to exert its calming influence.

The high road of the neocortex, specifically the medial prefrontal cortex (MPFC), has a difficult time countering the limbic system in threatening situations. In an untraumatized brain, the MPFC provides the feedback to shift the nervous system from the incited sympathetic fight-flight-fright response to the rest-digest mode of the parasympathetic nervous system. In a traumatized brain, neuroimaging scans show a propensity for decreased activity of the governing role of the MPFC and hyperactivity of the threat-detecting amygdala.[1]

What this looks like spatially is activation of the right hemisphere of the brain and a deactivation of the left. Later we'll explore these differences in brain laterality as they relate to trauma, contrasting procedural and declarative memory, but in short, the left hemisphere of the brain is more literal in its recall of events, while the right is more sensory and intuitive.

A child who has not yet learned to express themselves with

language relives trauma as bodily sensations and emotions. Neuro-imaging scans literally highlight this notion. What ensues with a traumatic flashback are the negative feelings without the capacity for rationalization. This begins the cascade of stress hormones that have long-term damaging effects on the body and promote cancer growth via several direct and indirect effects.[2]

While every human being experiences acute and chronic stress over the course of life, "stress hormones of traumatized people, in contrast, take much longer to return to baseline and spike quickly and disproportionately in response to mildly stress-ful stimuli," according to van der Kolk.[3]

PTSD patients experience this effect to the extreme when cortisol is elevated for such an extended period that the cells become numb to their influence. Cortisol dysregulation explains, in part, why chronic fatigue is a resultant and debilitating symp-tom of trauma.[4]

Research shows that mitochondrial dysfunction is associated with PTSD. As the energy generators of cells, anything that affects mitochondria can have damaging effects on metabolism. In a vicious cycle, once a metabolic deficit is initiated from a traumatic event, the resultant fatigue lowers resilience and the ability to respond to future stressful situations.[5]

Another feature evidenced by neuroimaging scans is that traumatic recall suppresses the thalamus, the key regulating struct-ure in the brain. The thalamus knits everything together: memory feeling, and rational interpretation. In the absence of that regulation, it becomes more difficult for the MPFC to reclaim healthy and calm nervous system function.

This all speaks to alteration in perception, but what about all the visceral symptoms experienced by trauma victims, particularly with preverbal trauma in young children? Neuroimaging of trauma patients also shows abnormal activation of the insula, a deep brain region that receives signals from the internal organs, muscles, and connective tissue.[6,7]

The insula is yet another brain region that can communicate a threat to the amygdala without input from the MPFC. If something doesn't feel right, that body sensation will cause hyperarousal long before the rational mind takes stock of the situation.

What we are talking about here is a set point for reactivity, where conditioned responses increasingly influence the behavior of the traumatized individual. This is the power of emotions, particularly negative ones. However, the brain is flexible, and it is possible to disengage long-standing negative responses and replace them with softer, well-adjusted ones. This is the promise of neuroplasticity.

The first step in that process is to differentiate between emotional states and traits. An emotional state is transient and situational. Picture being cut off while driving. An emotional trait is a conditioned response that repeats itself and becomes ingrained, which we then call a personality trait. While just about everyone will respond to being cut off with a temporary emotional state of agitation, a person with road rage is exhibiting an entrenched emotional trait.

Unpacking negative emotional traits is easier said than done, but it is possible using the techniques and therapies detailed later. What is germane to this discussion is that so many of our conditioned responses stem from past experiences, especially highly emotionally charged traumatic events. We make neuronal associations around those traumas—such as the world is an unsafe place —and those emotional traits continue to color our experience of the world until they are dismantled and replaced with a new belief. In other words, you must have a genuine and repeated experience of feeling safe in the world to counter the notion that the world is inherently unsafe.

A central tenet of neuroplasticity is that neuronal networks that fire together wire together. The brain can become adept at learning a new skill but can also become conditioned to feel unsafe as a habit. Our work is to calm the waters of the mind so the emotional mud of the past can settle. This restores clarity of thinking. From that clear place, we can once again see the true, peaceful depths of our being.

Adverse Childhood Experiences

With an appreciation for neuroimaging and neuroplasticity, it will be easier to connect the dots between trauma and cancer.

The Centers for Disease Control (CDC) and managed care consortium Kaiser Permanente collaborated with coprincipal investigators Robert Anda, MD, and Vincent Felitti, MD, to survey over 17,000 adults to understand the relationship between childhood trauma and incidents of disease and illness later in life. The data, collected between 1995 and 1997, became known as the Adverse Childhood Experience (ACE) Study, and its results suggest a strong connection between early childhood trauma and such disparate conditions as heart disease, substance abuse, and cancer.

Participants were asked to report the number of categories of trauma that applied to them instead of the number of incidents. The 10 ACE categories are:

1. Psychological abuse
2. Physical abuse
3. Sexual abuse
4. Emotional neglect
5. Physical neglect
6. Loss of a parent (for any reason)
7. Witnessing domestic abuse
8. Witnessing substance abuse of a close friend or family member
9. Mental illness experienced by a close friend or family member
10. Criminal behavior or imprisonment of a household member

The study found that upwards of two-thirds of participants surveyed reported at least one ACE, with about a fifth claiming three or more. All of these adverse experiences can disrupt normal psychological development in a child, giving rise to lifelong unhealthy behaviors like addictions as coping strategies. Stunted emotional maturity reinforces the notion that abuse and neglect perpetuate intergenerational trauma.

Even if child victims are successful in breaking the cycle in adulthood (for instance, refusing to hit their children despite the disciplinary beatings they received), that does not mean they are free from the trauma that may be unresolved in the heart and mind, festering its way into insidious physical and emotional disharmonies.

This may explain why the incidence for diseases such as cancer and heart disease goes up with every ACE a vulnerable youth undergoes. It's as if the seed of disease forms in a wound that hasn't healed, awaiting environmental factors to grow it into manifestation, be it a heart attack or a malignancy.

As researchers followed the progression of the ACE data, more telling trends have emerged. For instance, those with an ACE score of 6 or higher died almost 20 years earlier (on average) than those with a score of 0 and were twice as likely to be diagnosed with cancer.[8]

Research in the United Kingdom mirrors the findings of the American ACE Study. There, a five-decade study following thousands of participants from birth to middle age found that two or more adverse childhood experiences increased cancer risk two-fold in middle-aged women.[9]

The link is there; what remains is speculating the underlying mechanism(s) that drive illness in the presence of an ACE. Why does a history of trauma develop into one disease rather than another? I have two answers to this question, one for each side of the coin of epigenetics.

The most straightforward answer is toxicant exposure. In the presence of carcinogens and sluggish detoxification pathways, cancer is more likely to develop. Many chronic diseases such as cancer have genetic predispositions, but these genes are expressed under certain environmental conditions. The seed of cancer may very well be in all of us, but it only grows when the soil of trauma and bad weather of chemical carcinogens are present.

That is the external environment, but our internal environment is equally important. Thus, the other side of the epigenetics coin is a personality that is prone to cancer. That idea will take some unpacking.

Type C Personality

Medical psychology first postulated the theory that varying dispositions are predisposed to certain illnesses by defining a Type A personality. Impatient, competitive individuals who tend to overwork themselves are thought to be more prone to cardio-vascular disease.

In the late 1980s, psychologist Lydia Temoshok, PhD, started a movement to define a cancer-prone pattern of behavioral traits. According to the seminal research in this field, a Type C personality is "characterized by denial of negative emotions, inability to express feelings, and high social conformity and compliance."[10,11]

Other behavioral elements include shouldering others' burdens, struggling with healthy personal boundaries, and being a people pleaser. One hallmark of this type of pattern is internalizing emotions. Repression is unconscious emotional inhibition, while suppression is a conscious effort to do so. Neither is healthy, and although it goes against social norms in certain situations, with negative emotions, it is best for a Type C personality to express rather than repress or suppress.

Defining Type C personality traits came on the heels of older research, such as a 1982 study that showed a high correlation with malignant breast cancer biopsies in women prone to emotional suppression and avoidance of conflict. Interviewers of the patients and controls did not have access to biopsy results, and researchers based their designation upon interviews without contact with patients. It was a small study, but even so, a blinded rater could predict the correct diagnosis in 94% of all cancer patients and 68% of all benign cases.[12]

According to a 2000 paper, "Anger and Cancer," "There is evidence to show that anger can be a precursor to the development of cancer, and also a factor in its progression after diagnosis."[13] This includes prostate cancer in men, where anger suppression was significantly associated with decreased activity of natural killer cells, one of the key components of the immune system responsible for surveillance of rogue precancerous and malignant cells.[14]

While a behavioral pattern prone to cancer continues to be explored by the scientific community, it's not unreasonable to accept if we equate personality traits with constitution—a hallmark concept of traditional medicine that recognizes certain tendencies and behaviors favor the formation of one illness over another. For instance, someone with a hot constitution (yang excess in TCM) will have a ruddy complexion, forceful pulse, loud voice, and tendency toward agitation. These seem like minor observations, but collectively they frame what we now call a Type A personality.

There is nothing mysterious about constitution giving rise to illness. Seasoned medical providers can diagnose a patient long before performing confirmatory lab work. What we observe and label clinical intuition is probably the sum total of observations that infer a person's genetic and epigenetics factors, defined as one's phenotype in Western terms. Within that paradigm, not only is a "cancer personality" possible, it is diagnosable.

Now for the good news: Not only is constitution diagnosable, it is treatable. Whereas constitution and phenotype have inborn genetic characteristics, the epigenetic door swings both ways. Behavioral patterns are modifiable. Diet, lifestyle changes, meditation, etc., are well-established methods that hedge against inborn con-stitution and the associated behavioral traits.

That said, the notion of a Type C personality helps to frame our understanding of research, suggesting that trauma can change our internal environment and tip the scales toward cancer development.

Animal research from the 1980s studied how rats implanted with cancer cells can overcome the tumor burden based upon whether they are exposed to an inescapable trauma. The research-ers concluded: "Only 27 percent of the rats receiving inescapable shock rejected the tumor, whereas 63 percent of the rats receiving escapable shock and 54 percent of the rats receiving no shock rejected the tumor. These results imply that lack of control over stressors reduces tumor rejection and decreases survival."[15]

The artificial nature of this kind of research (implanting cancer cells) is not illustrative of how tumors form naturally in a rat, let alone a human being, but it makes you wonder how susceptible the disempowered and disenfranchised truly are in the face of ongoing trauma? If not a predisposing cause for cancer in-itiation, surely this must be a significant factor in relapse for a patient walking the razor's edge of remission.

Still, these effects may be relevant to us big-brained mam-mals, maybe even more so. Psychologist Martin Seligman, PhD, coined the term "learned helplessness" to highlight the effect of inescapable trauma, a notion shared by dissociation researcher Robert Scaer, MD, who relates helplessness and hopelessness to an unresolved freeze response.[16] Evidence linking adverse childhood experiences with disease, along with the possibility of a cancer personality, frame the broad psychosocial epigenetic factors that predispose cancer. Together with environmental carcinogen exposure, a strong case can be made that these epigenetic factors are more potent predictors of cancer than any combination of inherited genes.

This is the essence of traditional models of health and my personal philosophy of medicine. External disease factors include infections and toxin/toxicant exposure. Internal causes include stress and trauma. Revealing where those two meet—at the junction of human experience and perception—is the art of medicine.

While biomedical research continues the quest to elucidate the genetic underpinnings of cancer, realize that there are many epigenetic factors that are well within your power to change.

Environmental toxins, stress, and trauma are the elephants in the chemo room. Our bodies reflect the many forms of pollution that compose the carcinogenic soup we are all consuming.

But it's not always about what we are eating. Rather, it's about what is eating us. The poisons of guilt, fear, anger, anxiety, and depression result from traumatic experiences, and with them comes the propensity for cancer development. We'll come full circle to this idea in Chapter 7, but first we need to have a frank discussion on consciousness and the spiritual axis of being.

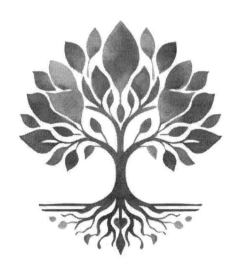

PART 2

Heart-Centered Consciousness

5

THE HARD PROBLEM OF CONSCIOUSNESS

"Consciousness is a singular of which the plural is unknown."

—Erwin Schrödinger, PhD

Nobel Prize-winning theoretical physicist

Any discussion of the origins and remedying of trauma must be viewed through the lens of perceptual awareness. The reason trauma reverberates through our being with its damaging influence lies in our perception of it. Trauma rarely occurs without a story being built around it.

We begin that discussion by exploring the subject of consciousness. The "hard problem of consciousness" proposed by philosopher and cognitive scientist David Chalmers, Ph.D., pertains to the subjective aspect of experience.

According to Chalmers in his book, *The Character of Consciousness:* "It is widely agreed that experience arises from a physical basis, but we have no good explanation of why and how it so arises. Why should physical processing give rise to a rich inner life at all? It seems objectively unreasonable that it should, and yet it does."

By contrast, the "easy problems of consciousness" are those that concern cognitive abilities and functions. To explain these phenomena, different models are posited, including the notion that aspects of consciousness arise from the peripheral nervous system, or even the organs, as is the TCM viewpoint. Another theory questions whether conscious awareness originates outside of the body, with the brain acting as a reducing valve, allowing certain experiences and excluding others. Let's explore these concepts to learn how they relate to topics such as emotions and intuition.

According to neuroscientist Paul D. MacLean's triune brain theory, the physical brain has three regions that are differentiated by its physiology. The brain stem controls involuntary mechanisms of life such as breathing and heart rhythm, the midbrain (limbic system) regulates emotions and memory, and the neocortex is associated with creativity and self-awareness. Together with the spinal cord, these brain regions compose the central nervous system.

The peripheral nervous system extends from the spinal cord to virtually every other part of the body, occasionally coalescing into dense networks called plexuses. The enteric nervous system is one such plexus centered around the digestive system, and the pneumogastric nerve connects the brain, heart, and gut.

In an example of bilateral communication, the intestinal microbiome of the gut produces the majority of the neurotransmitter serotonin that can be recruited by the central nervous system.[1]

The collective action of these functional relationships and anatomical structures has been called the gut-brain, and the communication between the enteric nervous system and the central nervous system is known as the gut-brain axis.[2,3]

Why have a gut-brain? Besides the obvious evolutionary advantage of having an intestinal awareness monitoring the health of all the foreign material passing through the digestive tract, there is also the verifiably real activation of a gut instinct. Indeed, many species that don't express higher brain functions survive due to the feedback provided by this ancient aspect of neurophysiology alone.

As every mother knows, instincts about the safety of one's children are exceedingly visceral. Triggered by stimulus recognition on the part of the central nervous system, the reactions within the gut-brain are the reason we feel "butterflies" in our stomach and why strong emotions can cause digestive problems with such conditions as irritable bowel syndrome.

The link between emotions and the nervous system of the gut is self-evident and was acknowledged long before neuroscience explored the connection. Suffice it to say, when working with strong emotions and trauma, the gut needs to be considered as a potential site of involvement.

I equate the gut-brain with subconscious awareness. As evolutionarily honed for survival as instinct is, I believe visceral sensations are the expression of intuition arising from the communications between the higher brain and the gut. When something feels right, beyond what is immediately apparent or even rational, that's gut instinct calling us to heed its old, intuitive wisdom.

Whether the physical brain is the seat of consciousness is an open-ended question, and adding the notion that aspects of consciousness reside in peripheral nerve plexuses, or even within individual cells, deepens that mystery. Cellular memory is a proposed explanation for phenomena that occur in only one part of the body.

Yet there is another aspect of consciousness that, although admittedly esoteric, is recognized by wisdom traditions of the indigenous world—the superconscious awareness of the human spirit. That the body either houses or expresses a superconsciousness has been the subject of philosophical and theological discussion for millennia.

It is challenging to avoid going too far down this rabbit hole when examining the presence or absence of the human soul or spirit solely through the lens of reductionist thinking; inevitably, one risks resorting to speculation. Instead, I will ask you to suspend preconceived reductionistic conclusions and consider the TCM model for superconscious awareness as a means to best understand the origins of emotions and how to heal from trauma.

In the TCM paradigm, there are five spiritual energies that inhabit the body, each an aspect of consciousness. Of those five, the spiritual energy of the Heart energetic has the closest resonance with what could be called a superconscious awareness. This essence, called "shen" in Chinese, is the spiritual aspect of oneself that receives inspiration from a greater source of awareness.

Note that the organs of TCM are functional descriptions, as opposed to anatomical. For example, the Spleen energetic is a placeholder for digestive function and all related organs, such as the stomach and pancreas. The TCM organ names are capitalized to distinguish them from the Western anatomical structure. We'll review the TCM organs and their emotional associations in a moment.

Whether superconscious awareness comes from some heavenly realm, deep neurocircuitry, or both is not of great concern in TCM. The Heart is the key to unlocking our greatest potential, and there is some fascinating science that illuminates this ancient observation.

Research by the HeartMath Institute has shown that the electromagnetic field of the heart extends farther from the body than the field emitted by the brain.[4] The pacemaker of the heart and related nerve bundles are highly active sensors of what is occurring in the blood, and that information is conveyed to the brain through afferent nerve fibers. In fact, more nerve signals travel from the heart to the brain than the other way around.[5]

The shen is the emperor of the governance of the body in TCM, and if we were to judge this declaration on the basis of the flow of information via the nervous system, the heart would dictate the lion's share of the discussion.

Thus, we have the TCM Heart as a third aspect of consciousness, one capable of contributing subtle information and inspiration to ordinary awareness, where it can be interpreted and made actionable. Now for the bait and switch: What TCM calls the shen of the Heart, I will now equate with the concept of the Heart-mind proposed in the introduction. The final axis may therefore be:

- neocortex-higher brain (conscious awareness)
- gut-brain (subconscious awareness)
- Heart-mind (superconscious awareness)

Subpersonalities

East Asian medicine isn't the only system embracing the fluidity of consciousness. In some branches of western psychology, it is theorized that different aspects of the self, known as subpersonalities, emerge when a person is under psychosocial stress. Richard C. Schwartz, PhD, introduced a therapy that takes advantage of this idea with Internal Family Systems. Alternatively known as the "Parts Work" model, as described by author Tom Holmes in a book of the same name, these therapies attempt to create an open dialogue with different aspects of one's self. Even if consciousness is singular, our experience of it is layered, thus a compartmentalized approach to awareness has a distinct psycho-therapeutic benefit.

Cognitive neuroscientist Michael Gazzaniga, PhD, has written extensively on the idea that the human mind functions as its own society. Gazzaniga's thesis is based on research with split-brain patients, who have a condition in which the corpus callosum is severed, preventing communication between the two hemispheres of the brain.[6]

Even without such an impairment, consider how mentally and emotionally divided we can be on a difficult subject. Maybe you have received a cancer diagnosis, and your head tells you to proceed with a conventional oncologist's plan of treatment, while your Heart-mind is siding with a contrasting plan offered by an integrative oncologist.

Moreover, there are parts of the human psyche that never stop perceiving developmental trauma as the child who experienced it, and that can be a very different perception from the adult viewing in retrospect. Whether subconscious or conscious, the child part feels despair, while the adult part responds with anger or violence.

Internal Family Systems derives its name from situations where different aspects of the psyche are akin to members of a family that have varied experiences and needs. In a psycho-therapeutic session, the client might be asked to have the angry part step aside and allow the abused child to voice what it needs to heal. This can be a profound intervention because a hallmark of trauma-induced dissociation is fracturing of the psyche. In therapy, Parts Work guides the client to witness these different aspects while cultivating mindfulness toward an undamaged essence, referred to as "Self," that can govern the reorganization of the parts to empower deep and lasting healing.

If this model of different parts of the psyche being viewed as family members sounds a lot like TCM's spirits of the organs—and specifically that the Parts Work term "Self" is akin to the shen of the Heart-mind—you are connecting some very important dots. Whether using the archaic but accurate language of spirits or the notion of parts that is more palatable to the Western mind, the concepts are quite similar in theory and application. As we will see, modern neuropsychology and ancient traditional medicine offer very different but congruous models for healing trauma.

6

THE HARD PROBLEM OF UNCONSCIOUSNESS

"When people under my care have died, I have often thought about the surface story of their death compared with what trauma was doing to them behind the scenes. This is nowhere more evident than in their listed cause of death. For example, the official version might be *car accident* as opposed to *raped by coworker*, or *suicide* instead of *swindled out of his life savings*, or *cirrhosis of the liver* in the place of *child abuse by alcoholic parent*. Trauma hijacks our stories in life and also in death."

—Paul Conti, MD, from *Trauma: The Invisible Epidemic: How Trauma Works and How We Can Heal From It*

A discussion of consciousness is incomplete without an examination of its antithesis, the cessation of consciousness as we know it. To heal from the trauma of cancer is to confront mortality. Cancer claims the life of many, leaving a wake of fear and despair in those left behind. There is no winning philosophy to address this existential fear. Instead, I favor reframing the conversation away from a mentality of preventing death toward an ethic of restoring life, love, and purpose.

First, it is helpful to distinguish between a fear of dying and a fear of death. The former is a process, while the latter is a state of being (or un-being, depending on your belief). For a cancer patient, the fear of dying is heavy with images of a body wasting away and riddled with pain. There is no way to sugarcoat this reality and the possibility of it happening following a cancer diagnosis. It's a terror all cancer patients must live with—or perhaps despite—the rest of their days.

Even if we cannot alleviate this fear, advances in compassionate medicine can still reduce its impact. There has been a shift in the paradigm of end-of-life care toward liberal use of hospice services and palliative care. The World Health Organization defines palliative care as "an approach that improves the quality of life of patients and their families facing the problem associated with life-threatening illness, through the prevention and relief of suffering by means of early identification and impeccable assessment and treatment of pain and other problems, physical, psychosocial and spiritual."

According to B.J. Miller, MD, author of *A Beginner's Guide to the End: Practical Advice for Living Life and Facing Death*, palliative care differs from hospice care in that the former is "patient- and family-centered care that optimizes quality of life and treats suffering. It is for anyone at *any* stage of serious illness, whatever the prognosis, and is intended to be delivered concurrently alongside other treatments, services, and primary care."

Miller clarifies that hospice care is a kind of palliative care "designed to treat physical, emotional, and spiritual discomfort for patients with a life expectancy of six months or less."

From this understanding, a hospice center is not a facility where one goes to die but a place of comfort to live well until one dies. That difference may seem subtle, but it is significant to cope with the psychological fear of dying.

As for the fear of death, few will arrive at their final moments without some regrets. As imperfect beings, we make many mistakes along the journey of life. Still, the fear of death can be softened. For an atheist, it may simply be the cessation of the suffering that can accompany the end of life. For those of faith, belief in an afterlife can lighten the burden of the unknown.

Cancer patient Anita Moorjani has a great deal to say about this topic in her book *Dying to Be Me*. As her organs were shutting down from a long and painful history with lymphoma, Moorjani slipped into a state of superconsciousness called a near-death experience (NDE). In that place, Moorjani describes her awareness as expanding to experience total love, acceptance, and peace.

From that place of superconscious awareness, Moorjani thought about the origin of her cancer and received a startling insight. She lived her adult life afraid that she would get cancer, and then it happened. She claims: "My many fears and my great power had manifested as this disease."

What happened next is as stunning as it is rare: She awakened from her NDE and started to heal. When before she had failed all lines of treatment, suddenly her therapy resulted in an extremely rapid shrinking of tumors in a well-documented case of spontaneous remission. Moorjani made a full recovery, is cancer-free, and travels the world sharing insights gleaned from her NDE. She isn't alone in her experience; thousands of such NDEs are cataloged by the Near-Death Experience Research Foundation.

Neurosurgeon and author of *Proof of Heaven*, Alexander Eben, MD, rapidly declined into a coma following a near-fatal bacterial meningitis infection when he, too, had a transpersonal NDE that radically changed his perception of reality. These experiences of an afterlife are different in the details but strikingly similar in the message gleaned. Both tell a tale of a total love and acceptance. Neither NDE contained dominant religious themes, which is poignant given Moorjani came from an Asian family with a Hindu upbringing, while Eben, Christian by upbringing but a professed atheist, was skeptical of spirituality before his NDE.

Another similarity in their accounts is the psychospiritual healing that occurred after the NDE. Both shared stories of traumatic experiences and profound healing that were informed by the consciousness shift inspired by their NDEs. Very few will have such dramatic paradigm shifts in consciousness as what Moorjani and Eben describe, but it is interesting to note how readily they connected their fears and traumas to impediments in daily living.

As Dr. Paul Conti conveys in the above epigraph, trauma is absent from a death certificate in a manner that underscores Western culture's inability to acknowledge how trauma "hijacks our stories in life and also in death." This is exactly why we need to shift our collective focus toward healing that which robs us of life even as we seek treatment to delay death.

The veracity of such NDEs is hotly debated, but the takeaway for me is singular. The Western mind is quick to position death as the opposite of life, but I view both dying and death as the process on the opposing pole of birthing and birth. Life has no opposite, similar to how physics posits that energy is neither created nor destroyed but only changes form. Energy, consciousness, life—they may all be different facets of the same eternal truth of existence.

Such a spiritual proposition may not be compelling or comforting to the cancer patient and caregivers in the midst of the death process. The mystery of consciousness will no doubt persist long into the future. Instead, I fall back on my roots as a biologist and rest in the truth that we are all part of a much larger process that has evolved over millennia. Seasons change, death gives rise to new life, and we all relinquish our bodies to an earth not inherited from our ancestors but borrowed from future generations.

Survivor Guilt

It is imperative to recognize that trauma can result from the cancer journey just as surely as it can predispose it. If undergoing conventional oncology treatment, the physical healing from surgery, chemotherapy, and radiation can take years; emotional healing can take even longer.

For a young parent, wrestling with one's mortality and the disruption to family life is potently traumatic. When I was diagnosed, my daughter was two years old. Although my wife and I tried our best to shield her from the worst effects, as time passed, we all exhibited symptoms of PTSD.

Then there's regret, shame, and guilt that can bubble to the surface. I remember the first time I experienced survivor guilt. I was speaking at a conference and caught up with a friend whom I had met at a previous event. Her young adult sister recently died of cancer, and she was candidly sharing her grief. I did not know her sister, but from keeping in touch in the years between, I had the impression that her sister was a beautiful soul with an easy smile and a compassionate heart.

Hearing the emotional retelling of the last days of my friend's sister and the traumatic fallout for the family was devastating enough. Having been in remission for a few years at that point, my empathy was raw and easily accessible. Yet I was unprepared for the level of guilt I experienced.

Why did this young woman succumb to cancer while I

endured? Did she access all the right treatments but not soon enough? Was it luck on my part? Should I, and could I, be happy amidst the wake of grief following her death?

At least I had an answer to the last question: Yes, I should live joyously, not despite this young woman's passing but because of it. It would be a disservice to her struggle and dishonoring of her memory to wallow in guilt while I had a family to nurture and patients to take care of. It didn't make the conversation with my friend any easier, but it softened the initial guilt that flooded my heart.

Survivor guilt can be a real obstacle for those in remission, especially when one reflects on younger individuals who die from a similar cancer that did not respond to the same treatment that led to their own remission.

Conventional medicine and the Western mind are ill-equipped to contextualize this paradox. Reductionist science may speak of a "success" or "failure" of treatment in terms of averages and proffer prognoses based on statistics, but that does little to ground the experience of each individual's cancer journey. There are almost 200 types and subtypes of cancer recognized by oncology, but I would argue that every case of cancer is unique, given the deep mental and emotional journey each patient has lived before diagnosis and will grapple with after remission.

As invested as I am in the power of mindset as an integral part of healing from cancer, I've seen some of the most upbeat, prayerful individuals die young from cancer. I've also observed some indifferent curmudgeons thrive against all odds. There is no secret formula for a healing mindset, save for total acceptance of any outcome, which also includes total acceptance of other cancer patients' responses to treatment.

If we are going to transcend the trauma inherent with cancer, we need to first accept it. This means considering cancer as a teacher and not an enemy. It means acknowledging that we may continue to get the lesson of cancer wrong for many more years—resulting in untold additional suffering—until a complete paradigm of integrative health ushers in a new model of treatment. That will take a monumental effort to bridge leading science and traditional wisdom but begins by accepting our vulnerability in the face of cancer and working through the grief that the word "cancer" conjures in the collective psyche of humanity.

I will give the last word to Rev. Tish Harrison Warren, who beautifully articulated human vulnerability in her book *Prayer in the Night: For Those Who Work or Watch or Weep*:

> The people who I most respect are those who have suffered but did not numb the pain—who faced their darkness. In the process they have become beautifully weak, not tough as nails, not bitter or rigid, but men and women who bear vulnerability with joy and trust. They are almost luminescent, like a paper lantern, weak enough that light shines through.

7

THE EMOTIONAL LANDSCAPE OF CANCER

"To completely heal a person, acupuncture, herbs, and these other modalities are only one aspect of the treatment. You must also come into synchrony with the patient in many other ways. For example, when patients lack the confidence to conquer illness, they allow their spirits to scatter and wither away. They let their emotions take control of their lives. They spend their days drowned in desires and worries, exhausting their essence, vital energy, and spirit. Of course, then, even with all these other modalities, the disease will not be cured."

—*The Yellow Emperor's Classic of Medicine*,
second century BCE

With a primer on consciousness in place, we can explore the role of the different TCM organs, the emotions associated with them, and how trauma can contribute to pathologies as complex as cancer.

In TCM, the primacy of health lies in the vigor of shen, the Heart-mind. Assessing the vibrancy of shen is fundamental to a practitioner of TCM. When consulting with a patient for the first time, I establish the strength of resolve to heal. Is the patient engaged, curious, hopeful? If so, the prognosis is good. For those who are depressed, defeated, or cynical, the prognosis may be poor.

Assessing shen takes into account a combination of verbal and nonverbal cues. The ability to hold eye contact and upright posture is an indication that the person's shen is strong, confirming the truth of their words. A mismatch between what a patient says and how the patient acts suggests an inner struggle or, at the very least, a lack of focus. This interpretation of shen is one aspect of mindset; the other aspects derive from the remaining spirits.

The Liver energetic contains the hun spirit, akin to what Western metaphysics defines as the astral body or soul. I think of the hun spirit as the dream consciousness giving rise to insight.

The Lung energetic houses the po spirit, or the etheric body. This is the energy body that TCM practitioners work with when performing acupuncture. This animate aspect is embodied at birth with the first inhalation and returns to the earth with our last exhalation at death. The expression of the po spirit is akin to the subconscious mind and, as previously discussed, experienced viscerally as intuition or gut instinct.

The Spleen energetic embodies the yi, or intention. By contrast, the Kidney energetic expresses zhi, often translated as will. I'll discuss these two together because of how they interact. Intention is baseless without the will to bring it to fruition. Likewise, having a strong will requires focused intention to produce any inner movement of value.

Putting it all together with an example, an insight is received from a dream (hun-Liver). Before being implemented, the idea should first have a clear sense of its "rightness." This is the confirming intuition (po-Lung) that sets intention (yi-Spleen) to work. That intention is the principle that requires the fuel of will (zhi-Kidney) to see it through. And the spirit of consciousness (shen-Heart) oversees it all, like an emperor on the throne, making sure every official is doing their job.

Taken collectively, the spirits of the organs frame the self as a thinking, feeling, willing, autonomous being. One need not believe in these spirits as metaphysical energies, particularly if the idea is unsettling or incongruous with one's religious beliefs. Taken metaphorically, the spirits represent different aspects of consciousness that seek alignment when healing from trauma. It is not enough to rally the thinking mind if one's gut instincts are telling a different story.

We can deepen our understanding of the different aspects of consciousness with the TCM emotional correspondence for each organ. The classics of TCM have a lot to say about the cause of disease that speaks volumes about the cancer epidemic. Most fundamentally, all disease arises from an imbalance with nature, or more specifically, from violations of natural law. That comes in many forms in an unhealthy, modern society: lack of sleep, a nutrient-poor diet, chronic stress, etc.

This sole principal of causality then splits into the yin and yang of disease etiology. Yang represents external pathogenic factors such as infections, physical trauma, and toxins. Yin represents an internal cause of a disharmony in the so-called seven emotions. If trauma is not about what happens to us but our internal response to it, then the TCM theory of the seven emotions is a roadmap to discover the breadth and severity of that response.

According to this concept, an emotional response to trauma does not affect the body uniformly—at least not at first. Of the five major organ systems, each has an emotion that tends to affect it more, with two organ systems having an additional emotional response associated with it. This brings the total to seven.

Note that this model is not written in stone, and any emotional disturbance can affect any one or more organ system. From clinical observation, they do tend to match up and can provide insight into the emotional underpinnings to cancer that originates in or near a specific organ.

Anger is the emotion associated with the Liver energetic and the Wood element. Frustration, rage, and generalized emotional stagnancy underlie a Liver-Gallbladder imbalance. This is an important emotional imbalance to start with for several key reasons.

Western culture is notorious for affecting Liver function. Be it the result of general stress from a fast-paced lifestyle or the many carcinogens that require detoxification, the modern human has more for the Liver to process than ever before.

In TCM, the Liver is the organ responsible for the movement of all emotions throughout the body. Stagnancy in the Liver can give rise to broad emotional volatility.

When the Liver is imbalanced, it then tends to "overact" upon the Spleen energetic. The diagnosis for this in TCM is Liver-Spleen disharmony and includes such symptoms and conditions as irritable bowel syndrome, premenstrual syndrome, fatigue, irritability, sleep disturbances, and many more. Liver-Spleen disharmony is the quintessential Western imbalance.

If left unresolved, anger can negatively affect Liver function and is associated with liver cancer. Disharmony between the Liver and Spleen due to suppressed, repressed, or overly expressed anger is associated with stomach, esophageal, gynecological, and pancreatic cancer. A right breast tumor can be associated with a Liver-Spleen disharmony when the Liver imbalance dominates.

When harmonious, the Liver energetic expresses perseverance, benevolence, and growth. This is anger and frustration mobilized to perform noble acts of service in the world.

For the Fire element of the Heart/Small Intestine energetic, the emotion associated with an imbalance is sometimes translated as joy or happiness. This doesn't quite tell the story. Excitement is closer, overexuberant is better still, and mania is the height of a Heart imbalance. Anyone who has witnessed an individual in the manic phase of bipolar disorder will have observed the emotional instability associated with the Heart.

There is nothing wrong with experiencing joy so long as it does not subjugate a core of calm. Excessive excitement scatters the Heart energy. Consider a child on Christmas morning, the internal fire of emotion burning so hot and bright that the red-cheeked youngling crashes in a tantrum as the excitement subsides.

If mania is the high-vibration extreme of an imbalance in the Fire element, the lower vibration emotional disharmony is anxiety. Although severe anxiety can be an overwhelming, whole-body experience, it tends to originate and radiate out from the center of the chest where the energetic Heart is situated. Those suffering from panic attacks often report palpitations as one common symptom.

Cancer associations include the heart and small intestine, lymphomas along the small intestine, and leukemia because of the connection of the Heart energetic with blood.

A balanced emotional expression of the Heart energetic is connection, community, and compassion. It represents our shared human experience, and the ability to lift one another up with an open heart.

Worry is the emotion that challenges the Spleen-Stomach energetic of the Earth element. Worry can manifest as a generalized angst or a fixation upon uncertainty, particularly as it relates to the future. A common aspect of worry is nervousness, as with an exam or job interview. A susceptible individual may find themselves running to the bathroom with acute gastrointestinal distress.

Another example is public speaking. Here, we can split hairs to showcase how emotions affect physiology. Although we often hear of the fear of public speaking, nausea experienced before performing is actually due to the Spleen and its connection to worry. Someone with a true fear of public speaking attempts to speak or perform and freezes in place. This is associated with the Kidney energetic.

All aspects of worry damage Spleen function and are associated with gastrointestinal cancers, left breast cancers, and lymphomas with spleen involvement.

The Spleen energetic is all about transformation and nurturing in its positive aspect. Free from worry, our ability to care for others as well as ourselves is the hallmark of a content and well-fed Spleen energetic.

The Lung/Large Intestine energetic of the Metal element has the two distinct emotional associations of grief and sadness. Grief carries with it regret or loss, such as when a close friend or family member dies, but can also be abstract, such as grieving a future that a cancer diagnosis has prevented. Grief strongly affects the Lung energetic. People exhibit grief through shallow breathing, a collapsed chest, and a hung head. It is as if the Lung energy is caving in under the weight of grief.

The TCM notion of sadness can also be translated as depression. It need not have an object of loss, as is often the case with grief. Depression can occur independent of circumstances and runs the gamut from feeling blue to severe clinical depression.

Associations with cancer include lung and large intestine malignancies, melanomas, and breast cancer in the upper lateral quadrant.

If the Spleen energetic is the mothering instinct, the Lung energetic expresses the ideals of fatherhood, honor, and value. The ability of the lungs to breathe deep and the colon to let go is the axis of the Lung and Large Intestine. While all emotions are "metabolized" by the Liver, the Lung plays a moderating role by helping the body-mind disperse and let go of any untoward emotion.

The Kidney-Bladder energetic of the Water element is the other organ system with two emotional associations: fear and fright. Fear differs from the uncertainty discussed with the Spleen. Fear of the unknown can manifest as dread and despondency. It is more debilitating than the worry associated with a Spleen imbalance.

The TCM conception of fright can also be translated as shock. This is the freeze response manifesting as dissociation. Trauma, at its core, is a challenge to the Kidney-Bladder dynamic and is also the startle response in mild form. When a person is scared to the point of "peeing their pants," that's the Bladder/fright connection.

It should come as no surprise that fear and fright are the dominant emotions associated with cancer when one's mortality hangs in the balance. Consider the shock following a diagnosis and the looming fear after being given a prognosis.

Direct cancer associations include kidney, brain, prostate, sarcomas, leukemias, lymphomas with bone marrow involvement, and metastases to the brain and bone.

A harmonious expression of the Kidney energetic is stillness and wisdom. Like a calm ocean deep with mystery, the ability to move through life with equanimity is the highest virtue of the Kidney energetic.

A disharmonious emotional response affects the body either through suppression or excessive expression. In the former instance, we suppress anger because it is not a socially acceptable time to air our frustration. In an example of the latter, fear can persist following the uncertainty of a cancer diagnosis.

The TCM notion of the seven emotions is meant to be an empowering treatise on health and well-being. If you notice a consistent disharmonious emotional response, whether suppression or excessive expression, consider the organ associated with that emotion. Once the organ is identified, take steps to practice its positive virtue to help heal that tendency. For example, fear can be softened by sitting in contemplative meditation, while anger's constructive outlet is benevolent service to others. Worry finds resolution in genuine care with good boundaries, not the burnout that caregivers so often experience.

Wood	Liver	Anger/Stress
Fire	Heart	Mania/Anxiety
Earth	Spleen	Worry/Nervousness
Metal	Lung	Grief/Depression
Water	Kidney	Fear/Shock

According to the Five-Element Theory of TCM, negative emotions can also be counterbalanced with the corresponding controlling emotion. The controlling cycle of the five elements is seen in the star pattern of the image. Wood breaks through Earth; Earth holds back the flow of Water; Water extinguishes Fire; Fire melts Metal; and Metal cuts Wood.

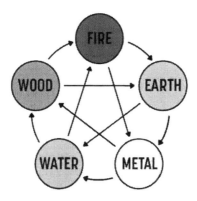

Here's an example of how to apply the principle of the controlling cycle: Inciting assertiveness as a healthy expression of the Wood element can pull someone out of persistent worry. Consider the cancer patient who breaks through worry like a seedling emerg-ing through the soil, becoming mobilized to action after a period of passivity. We leverage that assertiveness to create a vision for healing—that's the spiritedness of the Wood element correcting an Earth imbalance.

As another example, anger is often a mask obscuring unresolved grief. If an angry individual watches a sad film, tears may develop into weeping as the floodgates open. When empathy grants permission to cry cathartically, anger loses its rootedness. That's leveraging a beneficial expression of grief; the Metal element cuts through the aggression of Wood. This transformation is apparent in someone who says, "I was so angry, I cried."

Likewise, joy can assuage grief. In addition to honoring the dead, funerals bring the living together for mutual support. The Fire element of those in the community less affected by the loss helps warm the hearts of those deeply grieving. We offer a compassionate embrace or a shoulder to cry on, creating a safe environment for expressing grief.

The goal is not to become devoid of emotions, but to acknowledge their presence without judgment. By doing so, we allow the smooth flow of emotions through the body-mind, learn from them, and grow in virtue.

In the language of the classics of TCM, the character for emotion contains within it the notion of "that which is supposed to remain tranquil," whereas the character for virtue contains the attribute of "that which is meant to grow and reveal itself."[1]

The characters for emotion and virtue clue us in on how to do this: Find stillness within the torrent of emotion, and gain wisdom through the trials we face.

Coming full circle to the opening passage of this section, it is worth reiterating that in TCM, the primacy of health lies in the energetic Heart and the vibrancy of shen. The classic texts of TCM are clear in delineating the difference between stress and trauma. Acute stress affects the Liver whereas chronic stress depletes the body, causing a deficiency in Liver and Kidney function.

Trauma is diagnosed as Heart-shen disturbance in TCM. In Western terms, this is akin to stating that stress depletes the body and taxes the mind, but trauma fundamentally alters consciousness and inhibits spiritual expression—as is the case with dissociation. In this context, addressing trauma is a spiritual imperative.

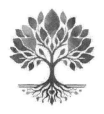

8

INTUITION AND INSPIRATION

"There is no such thing as a miracle which violates natural law. There are only occurrences which violate our limited knowledge of natural law."

—St. Augustine, fourth century CE

To close this discussion of consciousness, I want to expand on the notion that the body houses, at a minimum, three distinct aspects of consciousness and possibly more, as TCM upholds. Adding subconscious and superconscious awareness into the mix opens the door to intuition as a function of the former and inspiration of the latter. Let's compare those words to learn how to access subtle awareness as a healing force.

First, what is intuition and how do we experience it? This is a question I've thought a lot about as a practitioner of TCM. Though my work is based on the science of herbal prescribing and acupuncture point indications, there is also a subtle art to the medicine that draws heavily on intuition. After years of recognizing the flow of intuition, my interpretation is that one aspect of intuition is a subconscious conveyance of pattern recognition.

There is a scene in the 1988 film *Rain Man* in which Dustin Hoffman's character, an autistic savant, observes a dropped box of toothpicks and pronounces the exact number of strewn toothpicks. When he mutters the number 246, we are amazed by his extraordinary ability. But there's more to this scene than meets the eye, and that speaks volumes about what I think intuition is.

Consider how the brain works. To determine the total number of objects in a pile greater than ten or twenty, counting is necessary. Perhaps we count by twos or threes to quickly add up the total, but essentially we derive the solution by chunking, or breaking, the problem into smaller parts.

Chunking is not needed with fewer items because our brains can recognize a sum with a quick glance. If three pencils are on a desk, we don't count one, two, three. Instead, we see three items. If we're really good, perhaps we can register six or seven items. A mathematical savant would "see" 246 items as one complete perception. This is pattern recognition, and we do it all the time.

Reading an analog clock is a skill of pattern recognition. A digital clock displays numbers, and our brains interpret those numbers exactly. There is nothing ambiguous about seeing 4:24 p.m. on a digital clock. A child can easily tell time on a digital clock, yet understanding an analog one takes a little finesse. With learning to read an analog clock, the visual pattern of the hands provides more nuanced information because the part of the brain that processes spatial awareness also contributes to our sense of time. While the mathematical part of the brain is ascertaining the exact numerical time, the spatial aspect is providing a nonspecific interpretation of time.

Put another way, an analog clock need not have any numbers on its face, as with some wristwatches. The hatch marks that indicate the hour are sufficient for the spatial aspect of the brain to assess the approximate time with a quick glance. It is also easier to get a broader sense of time with a spatial awareness. Seeing a digital clock display 4:24 p.m. and recognizing that it is almost the half hour requires two steps: becoming cognizant of the exact time and then doing the math to see what fraction of the hour it is closest to. With an analog clock, we see the minute hand between the five and six and instantly know the time is almost 4:30. We can do this because of pattern recognition.

Now scale that ability to other aspects of life, and you'll see how intuition manifests. As a healthcare provider, I can often perceive an analogous thread in the symptom picture of a new patient that sparks a memory from someone I treated years prior. They may be totally different people, but something about the gestalt of their presentation matches, prompting me to connect the dots between how I treated the previous patient (if successful) and how I might care for the current patient.

What appears as intuition is not a conscious comparing of the two patients. As one fully formed thought, my brain made the connection and presented it to my conscious mind as a single coherent insight. This is the key to recognizing intuition. It doesn't arise as a stream of conscious thought the way we count items on a desk. Intuition is the ability to glance at a situation and get a mature assessment in a flash.

This brings up a few interesting points. First, nothing about this take on intuition is mystical. Pattern recognition is an innate feature of human evolution that aided our survival. We all experience eerie coincidences and serendipities, such as thinking of an old friend only to have that person call. I can't explain those, but the quality of everyday thinking gives rise to experiencing intuition almost daily.

Another point to consider is that intuition, as pattern recognition, is a feature of subconscious cognition. When our thinking mind evaluates a situation, it occurs in our native language; we literally speak to ourselves with the syntax of language. When we experience intuition, it is a subconscious awareness that arises as a feeling, impression, or state of knowing, without being bound by words. This is what we do when we look at an analog clock and what Dustin Hoffman's character did when he saw the box of toothpicks fall—we gauge the situation as a cohesive whole.

Life experience helps us cultivate intuition. The more general knowledge we have on a subject, the better equipped we are to receive intuitive impressions about it.

The other key element to developing intuition is letting go of conscious perception and allowing the body's innate wisdom to speak. This is easier said than done, but the eye perceives and the body feels way more than what filters into our conscious experience. What remains in the recesses of the subconscious is the basis for intuition as pattern recognition. Any mindfulness practice that calms the thinking mind in deference to the feeling body can help spark intuition.

The last step is to practice letting these moments speak to you. When preparing a meal, can you glance at a pantry shelf, as with an analog clock, and feel what would best nourish your body-mind? Or, can you reflect on myriad symptoms from seemingly disconnected health problems and derive a casual pattern? If so, you've just flexed your intuitive muscle and are one step farther down the road of personal empowerment.

৽৵৶

If intuition is a subconscious rendering of insight born of innate intelligence, inspiration is a superconscious opening to infinite intelligence. Whereas the former is grounded in our primal gut instinct, the latter is an expression of a higher mind.

Being connected to a universal stream of consciousness may sound as unattainable as it is mystical, but doing so is an inherent feature of a broader spiritual reality we share. From pre-civilized shamanic peoples to modern spiritual traditions, the same theme has echoed across millennia: We are not human beings having spiritual experiences but spiritual beings having human experiences.

Acknowledging a spiritual dimension to existence is not prerequisite to experiencing inspiration but it is helpful for its cultivation. (After all, you rarely find what you are not looking for.) Sometimes an insight smacks into our oblivious consciousness as an act of divine grace, but more often it percolates to the surface during periods of introspection.

Therein lies the key to cultivating inspiration, calming the mind of ordinary thought long enough for extraordinary insight to arise. The difference between intuition and inspiration is this: Intuition arrives as a polished flash of insight, while a deep emotional charge accompanies inspiration. Intuition comes as a knowing; inspiration is a knowing combined with a feeling, be it peace, wonder, or a sense of rightness. Sometimes that feeling is so powerful that it becomes a preoccupation. Consider the artist or inventor who gets a new inspiration and becomes laser focused on it, neglecting sleeping and eating until the vision is preserved.

The root of "inspiration" is "inspire," and this gives us a clue as to how a spiritual insight becomes embodied. In TCM, the concept of qi (often translated as vital energy) literally means "breath" or "air." This has several implications. One way to bring energy into the body is through the physical act of respiration, but we also "breathe in" spiritual insight.

TCM has long upheld that humans are amalgamations of heaven and earth. We combine yang energy (spirit) from above with yin energy (body) from below to form an existence that interfaces between the two worlds. As the qi of heaven is metaphorically represented as air, we breathe in spiritual insight throughout life.

We can also collectively channel inspiration into human consciousness. Whether via group prayer or a think tank, when we conspire (etymologically, to co-inspire, meaning breathe together), we create a flow of energy toward a shared goal. What we conceive as brainstorming is often a tapping into universal consciousness to derive unique insight.

Eureka moments punctuate life, but the quality of everyday inspiration is an insight that feels right. As a clinician, I aim to predispose inspiration within a therapeutic relationship. A problem that clinicians and patients alike face is not knowing what you don't know. A detailed case history will fill chart notes with relevant information about how and when an illness develops but may not elucidate the why. As Albert Einstein is often quoted as saying, "No problem can be solved from the same level of consciousness that created it."

Sometimes we need inspiration to derive the proper course of action. It is a beautiful moment to behold when the clinician reflects upon a patient's story and an "aha" moment alights both faces. I'll never forget one such moment.

A patient presented with acute sciatica, a shooting nerve pain from the hip down through the leg. When asked what was happening around the time the problem started, the patient responded that she was preparing to attend a family gathering. I notated this and later in the intake inquired about general stresses in the patient's life. She commented on a falling out with her father a few months prior. I set this piece of information aside until later when an insight flashed into my consciousness like lightning.

I asked if this family gathering would be the first time seeing her father since the estrangement. Her demeanor shifted as the lightning bolt struck her next—indeed, it was an unsought re-union. I elaborated on the psychospiritual metaphor of the sciatica. She was attending the gathering due to a sense of family obligation, but her body was literally trying to prevent her from walking toward her father. As should be clear by now, trauma often manifests somatically; we carry our issues in our tissues.

This association may be coincidence, but consider the course of resolution for this patient's condition. She responded favorably to acupuncture with a marked reduction in pain, but the problem did not resolve until she healed her relationship with her father. One day she came to her appointment without pain, describing with great emotion the forgiveness that occurred between them.

When I saw this patient in the future, she reported that her sciatica never returned. I can't take credit for that, save for being a mirror of the patient's experience and conveying an inspiration for the root cause of her discomfort. This wasn't intuition subconsciously assembled from pattern recognition; it was an inspiration about a causality that I could not rationally know.

Whether one is deep in meditation or out for a long walk, inspiration can arise when it's not expected or be rallied by spiritual forces to predispose it. The key is to first realize the possibility and open oneself to experiencing inspiration. Then, when an insight occurs, notice how you feel as much as what you are thinking. Does the insight bring with it a feeling of inner peace and alignment that resonates with every fiber of your being? If so, make the most of the opportunity to bring the insight into fruition.

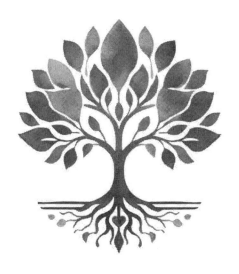

PART 3

A Path to Healing

Generally speaking, there are two ways to work with trauma. The first approach focuses on indirect methods that build resilience and instill a general sense of calm. Several of these strategies were explored in depth in my book *Cancer, Stress & Mindset* and include such practices as meditation and optimizing sleep. Although helpful for raising the set point for stress resilience, many of those strategies can directly address traumatic memories with a therapist's guidance.

Directly confronting trauma aims to desensitize the specific feelings, emotions, and associations of a traumatic event. Here, we can divide therapies into two categories. Somatic therapies emphasize the body, unconscious processing, and resolving implicit procedural memories of trauma. Cognitive therapies tie in executive functioning in the brain to downregulate arousal of the amygdala and leverage explicit declarative memory to oust traumatic images and sensations. If those concepts are foreign, you'll clearly understand what they mean by the end of this section.

Whether the approach used is top-down (cognitive) or bottom-up (somatic), addressing trauma directly is not without its challenges. For starters, deep-seated trauma often gets suppressed for a reason, and few should dredge up the past without the guidance of a qualified mental health professional.

For this reason, it is prudent to first practice indirect methods of building stress resilience while establishing a healing team. What you don't want is to dive headfirst into trauma resolution without having a system of stress management in place. While trauma work restores agency, it is possible to be more in control of your narrative and still be hyper-aroused, a state that Alcoholics Anonymous calls "white-knuckle sobriety."

The converse is also true when desensitization does not lead to integration. Cancer patients may be offered several avenues of counseling or group therapy for guidance on managing the stress of a cancer diagnosis, but these resources may not be adequate to process developmental trauma. Because conventional medicine is hesitant to associate past trauma with present illness, trying to connect those dots in a cancer support group may fall on deaf ears. The strategies presented here are an exploration of options that will require follow-up with the appropriate health care provider. When assembling a healing team, an ideal advocate is one with whom you feel safe to address the many layers of trauma. I cannot emphasize this point enough; the therapeutic relationship is primary. Compassionate engagement from a health care provider may be the single best predictor of success with any intervention.[1]

Any one therapy, skillfully applied, has the potential to be effective. According to a University of Wisconsin meta-analysis comparing the relative efficacy of various psychotherapies for PTSD, the authors concluded that compared to no therapy, "bona fide psychotherapies produce equivalent benefits for patients with PTSD."[2]

What therapy or therapies you choose will depend on access and cost. When considering these strategies, leverage intuition for what feels right, and take the path of least resistance. There are many helpers; find the one(s) who can bring you home.

Before we start a detailed discussion of strategies to integrate traumatic experiences, I would like to write a few words for caregivers and supporters who are not trained trauma therapists. If someone close to you has been diagnosed with cancer and is in a state of shock, please listen carefully to this message: The existential crisis from a life-threatening diagnosis can be all consuming, just when decisions about one's care require an inward focus. And that's the unfortunate reality—the trauma of cancer pulls us out of our body at the exact time we need to be fully rooted in it.

There is a flurry of activity during the initial weeks following a cancer diagnosis, beginning with a battery of testing to solidify the diagnosis. This is followed by treatment recommendations, which often include a second or third opinion supplemented with all the research Dr. Google can muster. Self-care isn't the obvious priority at this stage, but taking the time to cultivate an anticancer mindset means having access to all our faculties—body, mind, and spirit—to foster the best possible outcome.

Although the onus for accessing that state of being rests solely on the individual, caregivers can play a key role in influencing the likelihood of success. The virtue that best exemplifies the role of the supporter can be described with one word: authenticity. What that entails requires a bit of explanation.

Authenticity for a health care provider or caregiver is composed of three interdependent qualities. The first is the ability to be present with another human being while that person struggles. This means not being distracted, listening with an open Heart-mind, and seeing the process from start to finish on the patient's timeline. This is rarely possible for a health care provider who has a limited amount of time to interact with a patient. That's where social workers, therapists, clergy, family, and friends can all help, providing dedicated and focused attention to allow a healing mindset to arise.

The second quality of authenticity is veracity. For those un-familiar with the word, it denotes truthfulness but with an emphasis on sincerity. Sometimes being honest about a difficult situation means not painting a rosy picture in the face of a serious cancer diagnosis while at the same time not being overly focused on the drama of the challenge. Veracity entails meeting people where they are at and not trying to change the narrative if it is uncomfortable. Being a witness to traumatic events is difficult. Caregivers have to draw on their own inner-development work to avoid burnout.

This brings us to the third quality of authenticity—compassion. The human experience is a tribal one. We are social mammals living within communities, having developed a nervous system with mirror neurons that enables us to experience empathy. We bear wit-ness to each other's struggles while reflecting upon our own, hope-fully doing so from a grounded and objective place. When someone is deep in a metaphorical hole (whether by circumstance or self-inflicted) it is of no help to jump in with that person. Compassion is throwing down a rope with your feet firmly planted. It's empathy with healthy boundaries.

Together, these qualities of presence, veracity, and com-passion frame the virtue of authenticity. In a perfect world, every contact with medical or mental health professionals would em-body these principles. Sadly, that isn't always the case. Diseases such as cancer evoke much fear and remind us of our mortality. The cancer journey can be a traumatic one, to say nothing about the mental, emotional, and spiritual backdrop of the person receiving the diagnosis. At the intersection of past trauma and fear of the future is the precarious position in which the caregiver is placed. But if poised with authenticity, the caregiver can be a beacon of light during a dark time.

9

THINKING THROUGH TRAUMA

"The unexamined life is not worth living."

—Socrates

Psychotherapy

Perhaps no one better understands what it means to move through the pain of trauma toward wholeness than Holocaust-survivor-turned-psychiatrist Viktor Frankl, MD. In his celebrated book *Man's Search for Meaning*, Frankl describes the existential vacuum of searching for the meaning of life and suggests three ways of finding purpose in his psychotherapy approach, known as logotherapy. The first is through dedication to one's work, particularly in a creative endeavor. Artists of every type can experience a profound summoning of life force through creative expression.

The second is in relationship with others through love. Whether raising a family or compassionately serving others, as exemplified by the work of the late Mother Teresa, connection within communities and the natural world places our purpose within a larger, externalized context.

The third way to find meaning in life, according to Frankl, is the path of suffering. He reflects specifically on the plight of a cancer patient in his writing: "When we are no longer able to change the situation—just think of incurable disease such as in operable cancer—we are challenged to change ourselves."

That's easier said than done. This third path of suffering is unquestionably the hardest to derive meaning from when thrust into the psychological torrent of facing one's mortality, managing symptoms from the disease and the side effects of treatment. If Frankl can survive years of being starved and tortured to near death within a concentration camp, then there is hope for those of us dealing with the aftermath of a cancer diagnosis.

William Breitbart, MD, is the chair of the Department of Psychiatry and Behavioral Sciences at Memorial Sloan Kettering Cancer Center. Breitbart grew up in a community of Holocaust survivors and is the son of parents who endured trauma and conflict during the war.

In addition to the circumstances of his upbringing—or perhaps because of it—Breitbart was diagnosed with thyroid cancer at 28. Although he was cured, the vulnerability of his health crisis persisted. That experience inspired him to develop a program in meaning-centered psychotherapy to address the psychological fallout from cancer.

Breitbart was finding a profound despondency in advanced cancer patients, with some to the point of giving up on all future happiness. In the experienced eyes of Breitbart, these patients had lost meaning, and giving meaning to the rest of their lives became his method of helping them transcend their suffering.

Like Frankl, Breitbart posited that we must create meaning from our trials. Among the core principles is to focus on what is quintessentially you, separate from identifying as a cancer patient. With the tools of psychotherapy, Breitbart successfully brought cancer patients back from the depths of their existential despair, and research on meaning-centered psychotherapy has proven it to be an important tool to help patients stuck at the intersection of trauma and cancer to heal.[1,2]

From Chapter 2, you may recall that the research literature shows evidence of a transgenerational effect of trauma, and I hinted that healing can also be transmitted. Results of a 2013 study published in *Frontiers in Psychiatry* suggest that psychotherapy can produce positive epigenetic changes in combat veterans.[3] In other words, if a traumatized individual does the work of healing from the past, the effects of that trauma need not affect future generations. Positive psychotherapy can undo the effects of trauma on an epigenetic level.

Recall the animal studies with traumatized mice passing along erratic behavior to their offspring. Mansuy's team performed additional research on an epigenetic healing effect and found that traumatized mice, given a nurturing environment of safety and activity, did not pass on distressing behavior to their progeny.[4]

All this is to say that there are a lot of levers of healing that can be pulled, and the process need not be formally conducted by a psychotherapist. Whereas working through highly charged emotional experiences is often best done with a trusted and compassionate therapist, it is possible to conduct self-guided therapy sessions.

A few months after my cancer diagnosis, I made a recording where I talked myself through several childhood and recent traumas. Although they were upsetting times in my life, recalling these memories was not overwhelming. Thus I felt safe journaling the details of these incidents after a deep meditation session.

This "emotional-moments" exercise is loosely based upon a guided reflection from the book *Mind Over Medicine: Scientific Proof That You Can Heal Yourself.* In a chapter titled "Radical Self-Care," Lissa Rankin, MD, guides readers to discover their intuitive voice, what she calls our "Inner Pilot Light," in order to write "The Prescription" for wholeness in every aspect of life: physical, mental, emotional, financial, relational, etc.

A comprehensive evaluation of the direction of one's life can be a heart-wrenching exercise when brutal honesty forces the realization that "My job is killing me" or "My marriage has been over for years." These are not comfortable truths, but they are truths requiring examination if we are to translate the symptoms of our body into motives of healing. Not doing so—only seeking a cure while forsaking a return to wholeness—risks not addressing the root cause of illness.

With cancer, we can successfully shrink tumors using drugs or excise them from the body with surgery. Yet this question remains: Have we grown more empowered by doing so? Introspection is medicine, and examining the trajectory of our lives with an eye toward wholeness is the promise of positive psychology.

Frankl reflects upon his experience in a concentration camp with what I believe to be the ultimate goal of introspection. In his own words:

… It did not really matter what we expected from life, but rather what life expected from us. We needed to stop asking about the meaning of life, and instead to think of ourselves as those who are being questioned by life—daily and hourly. Our answer must consist, not in talk and meditation, but in right action and in right conduct.

Meridian Tapping

The combination of Western psychotherapy and TCM principles has given rise to a modality called meridian tapping. I first learned of and practiced a predecessor therapy called Emotional Freedom Techniques (EFT), developed by Gary Craig, in the 1990s. In essence, it combines affirmations with tapping on acupoints to free the body of physical and emotional pain.

Its earliest use was with phobias, tapping acupuncture meridian points while calling to mind a scene that elicited hyperarousal. The results for this application were dramatic, often with a single session of reframing affirmations resolving a fearful response to phobias that persisted for years.

The next generation of therapists experimenting with EFT soon discovered that it worked well for chronic pain, especially discomfort that began insidiously without a precipitating physical trauma, or intermittent pain that worsened when under mental or emotional duress. This recalcitrant form of chronic pain that is linked to traumatic events is called neuroplastic pain. It is thought to derive from sensory neural circuits in the brain that continue to activate when stressed or with the recollection of trauma. Therapists practicing EFT discovered that they could grant their clients relief from the physical and emotional fallout of long-standing trauma.

EFT became refined into a smaller subset of techniques and is now simply known as meridian tapping. The key to success with meridian tapping is to leverage affirmations that conjure the emotion of a traumatic event to release the trauma from the energetic anatomy of the acupuncture meridians. The physical action of tapping on acupoints signals the governing action of the brain to rapidly process the traumatic experience.

Where there was a memory with an intense emotional charge, tapping with affirmation dissolves the charge until only the memory remains. This is an important point. Nothing short of amnesia removes the memory of trauma. Instead, therapies like meridian tapping guide the consciousness of the individual to a safe place where the trauma can be viewed without the physiological fallout of PTSD symptoms. Thus the results of meridian tapping are not an end in and of themselves but the means to begin the healing process by removing the energetic disruption associated with trauma.

For this, meridian tapping is a gift that works beautifully under the guidance of a skilled therapist. It's curious to think that meridian tapping exerts its influence via stimulating acupuncture points. As a licensed acupuncturist of many years, I can attest that acupressure, whether by massage or tapping, can elicit a significant activation of the nervous system.

Another aspect is that statements of affirmation and mechanical stimulation may condition the prefrontal cortex to override the limbic-system when recalling a traumatic memory. Whatever the case, there is research evidence showing that meridian tapping improves multiple physiological markers, such as resting heart rate, blood pressure, and cortisol levels. The most impressive effect documented was an alteration in gene expression, the bedrock of hardcore Western biomedicine.[5,6]

A 2012 study in the journal *Traumatology* showed that even a single session of meridian tapping reduced the intensity of traumatic memories in abused adolescents compared to the control group that did not receive treatment. Perhaps any intervention involving human attention would cause some beneficial change when compared to no intervention, but keep in mind that not all therapies that dredge up traumatic memories are successful. Haphazard trauma therapy can increase anxiety, so even a pilot study of a single intervention that shows efficacy is noteworthy.[7]

Meridian tapping is one of many techniques under the umbrella of energy psychology. Similar to acupuncture, meridian tapping's strength is in its subtlety, drawing upon the innate healing potential of accessing the heart-mind-body connection. The technique differs from acupuncture in its use of affirmations to highlight the origin of distress. For example, an affirmation surrounding a trauma may be worded, "Even though I get anxious driving through the intersection where I had my accident, I deeply love and accept myself."

This presents a unique benefit in leveraging the combined forces of the conscious and subconscious aspects of awareness. Using language to tie thoughts with emotions and visceral sensations, meridian tapping offers a gestalt approach to psychotherapy.

Eye Movement Desensitization and Reprocessing

From Chapter 2, you may remember that trauma leaves a visceral impact, and the brain stores it as procedural (unconscious, long-term) memory. This is especially true of traumatic events occurring to a child who has not mastered language. Eye movement desensitization and reprocessing (EMDR) is one of several therapies that attempt to shift traumatic memories away from procedural storage into declarative storage, where rational processing occurs in the brain. This is a top-down approach in which conscious awareness can reframe traumatic events from a safe and clear place.

Psychotherapist Francine Shapiro developed EMDR in the 1980s when working with PTSD patients to help identify and process traumatic memories and their negative associations related to thoughts, judgments, and emotions.[8]

At its core, EMDR works by providing bilateral stimulation of the senses. Historically, this was done by the therapist waving two fingers back and forth in front of the patient's eyes. This metronome-like visual cue aims to free the traumatic "target," as EMDR calls it, through short-term, or working, memory.

To get a sense of the clinical application, I spoke with licensed professional counselor and trauma specialist Deb Meisner, who practices EMDR for processing trauma. A seasoned therapist, she embraces the next generation of EMDR technology that uses a customizable computer program combining alternating auditory cues and a visual stimulus. She prefers the visual setting that displays a lemniscate pattern.

Traumatic dissociation can predominate in one side of the brain in procedural memory, where it is nonverbal and somatic. According to Robert Scaer, MD, in his book *The Body Bears the Burden*:

… Positron emission tomography (PET) studies in arousal activation in PTSD patients suggest a significant lack of physio-logical coherence between the cerebral hemispheres in patients with PTSD. Several studies using quantitative EEG (QEEG), and single photon emission computerized tomography (SPECT), also support this concept of impairment of cerebral hemispheric synchronicity in PTSD, and show preliminary evidence for integration and reactivation of metabolically inhibited regions in the left hemisphere by relatively brief treatment with EMDR.

It's unclear whether traumatic dissociation is the cause or result of this lack of coherence in the brain, and possibly both are occurring in a vicious cycle. Whatever the case, many therapies that address trauma rely on movement or expression that engages both sides of the brain. For EMDR, alternating bilateral stimu-lation while focused on the traumatic target moves the memory to declarative memory, where all aspects of the brain can integrate the experience.

Meisner conducts therapy sessions in person or through a telehealth platform, guiding clients through traumatic memories with a remote EMDR computer application. Her process always begins with resourcing, a theme that comes up in many therapies addressing trauma. Resourcing is a resilience-building strategy that creates a positive buffer to prepare for tackling the negative thoughts, feelings, and emotions associated with trauma.

Clients are actively led through a visualization process to

create a container where they can lock away negative impressions. Details are important. While the container can be made of any material, attention must be given to the type of lock and how it operates. The container can change size as needed, but items placed within can never escape. There is also the assurance that the imagined container belongs only to the client, and no one else can ever access it.

Placing negative thoughts or feelings into the container is one technique of many that comprises what Meisner calls a mental first-aid cabinet. With these or other resources in place, EMDR sessions can then proceed to identifying a target, rating its level of discomfort on a scale of 1 to 10 (with 10 being the most distressful), and then using repeated rounds of bilateral brain stimulation to slough off the negative association of the trauma with the goal of reaching 0.

Not all clients respond well to the standard visual and audio cues. For those with visual or hearing impairments, a kinesthetic stimulus is used to create the bilateral point of focus. This can include tapping each side of the body in an alternating fashion.

When addressing severe trauma, EMDR therapists may need to use multiple bilateral stimulation approaches to strongly activate working memory. A patient might be asked to move their body while focused on alternating visual and auditory cues. This suggests that EMDR does indeed leverage working memory to oust the various negative associations with trauma.

Think of it this way: Deep procedural memory of trauma is a

subconscious impression. To this gray sketch of a traumatic event, the limbic brain adds its color. Perhaps there is a judgment, such as self-blame for abuse. Or maybe the connection is visceral, and the sensation of emptiness in the pelvic region adds a somatic element to the memory.

In all these cases, layers of associations prevent trauma from being processed by declarative memory where the rational regions of the brain can positively reframe them. In an EMDR session, focus on the target dredges up all the negative thoughts, feelings, and emotions associated with the trauma. But instead of trying to talk though it, the focus shifts to recalling the traumatic experience while running through rounds of bilateral brain stimulation. And then, by some magic, while the brain is receiving a multitude of bilateral stimulation, the negative charge surrounding the trauma is gradually liberated from the memory itself.

Thus, the short-term nature of working memory bridges the two forms of long-term memory: implicit/procedural memory and explicit/declarative memory. Practically speaking, this means the recall of a trauma never goes away; one can't simply erase the recollection of a painful event. Instead, the traumatic memory, now a resident of declarative memory, can be reflected upon and discussed without all the negative associations that accompanied it in procedural memory.

Neuroscience may reveal that everything described in the last few paragraphs is imprecise at best or outright wrong at worst. What matters is that many people struggling to overcome trauma have found benefit from EMDR, and clinical research supports this assertion. One study suggests that EMDR is at least equivalent and sometimes superior to antidepressants in relieving symptoms associated with PTSD.[9]

One limitation of EMDR revealed in that study (similar to other top-down approaches) is addressing childhood abuse, where somatic symptoms predominate in the absence of a rational narrative. It appears EMDR is best positioned to affect PTSD in trauma experienced as an adult, but some clinicians disagree.

Sandra Paulsen, PhD, published a book, titled *When There Are No Words: Repairing Early Trauma and Neglect From the Attachment Period With EMDR Therapy*, with specific guidance to address somatic distress. EMDR is actively being used to treat pre-verbal trauma.

In a 2013 guidelines document, the World Health Organization recommends that "individual or group cognitive behavioral therapy (CBT) with a trauma focus, eye movement desensitization and reprocessing (EMDR) or stress management should be considered for adults with posttraumatic stress disorder (PTSD)."[10] The quality of evidence for both CBT and EMDR is rated as moderate.

How movement of the eyes can drive neurological changes brings up a curious observation on the evolution of vision. The eyes of most predators (humans included) face forward to provide binocular vision, while prey animals tend to have eyes situated toward the sides of their heads to optimize peripheral vision. The hormone signature of a heightened stress response, epinephrine and norepinephrine, causes the eyes to deviate outward and the pupils to dilate to scan the environment for threats. This is an autonomic response. If the stress spills over into a freeze response without subsequent resolution, this ocular divergence can become an ingrained pattern, resulting in binocular dysfunction.

Put another way, humans are evolved to be hunters with clear and sharp binocular vision. With dissociative trauma, the focus of the visual field shifts outward as if the person has become an animal hyperalert to predation.

This makes me wonder about early childhood trauma and a subtle impairment in the proper functioning of the eye muscles that predisposes nearsightedness. That might be a hard sell for a conventional ophthalmologist, but a more typical pattern is for a traumatized individual to experience tunnel vision with repeated duress. I had this problem for many years. When in a very uncomfortable situation, my vision would change, and everything would seem far away. It was as if my brain was trying to separate myself from the environment, even when my body couldn't escape.

Whether my observations are characteristic of a larger connection between trauma and alterations in vision remains to be seen. Regardless, therapies like EMDR leverage healthy, bilateral movement of the eyes to safely resolve trauma.

ADDRESSING TRAUMA WITH EMDR

After interviewing Deb Meisner, I scheduled an appointment to experience EMDR. We spent the first portion of the session developing my container and exploring a peaceful place within my imagination. The latter came easily from years of practicing shamanic journeying, during which I almost always begin the experience from my inner peaceful place in nature.

The building of a container was a new concept, and I used my powers of imagination to define every detail of the iron-bound oaken chest that was to be my personal dumping ground for unwanted thoughts and emotions. As instructed, I placed special attention on the character of the lock and key, committing to memory every detail of how this connection point was to be made unassailable.

In my experience, details like these strengthen the mental exercise of any visualization practice. The more you can convince yourself of the importance of an image, the more real and valuable it becomes. Then, when presented with an opportunity to liberate negative energy into the container, it is easier to feel its power as much as see it in your mind's eye.

To strengthen the metaphor of a locked container, Deb offered that anything cast within the container would be irrevocably frozen in place. I found this notion appropriate, given trauma's ability to freeze the body and mind with dissociation. To freeze away that which binds is a clever way to transfer trauma and empower the healing process.

My take on this freeze-in-place imagery was slightly different. Being a child of the '80s, I couldn't help but picture my container sucking in negative energy like the ghost traps from the film Ghostbusters. With that image in mind, I took a few minutes to dump some recent stresses (the ghosts of my psyche?) into the chest for permanent containment. Feeling lighter, I spent some time in my peaceful place preparing for the next phase of the work. After each of these exercises, the EMDR program was used to run one cycle of alternating visual and auditory stimuli to integrate the work.

The second half of the session focused on the alleviation of one target that I had planned to address when I made the appointment. A recent trauma in our family still weighed heavily on me, so when I was asked what I wanted to work on, I explained the basics of the story with enough information to be guided through the process but not enough detail to risk becoming too upset to proceed. This was per Deb's request, not only to keep me comfortable but also to avoid burdening her with the full emotional content of my experience. Being a therapist is hard work, and I imagine the job comes with a high burnout rate. Keeping the dialogue focused but not evocative dissuades the transference of trauma.

After establishing the target, the EMDR program was set with different alternating visual and auditory stimuli. Although similar in their deployment, one contrasting pattern is designated for positive reinforcement, while the other is reserved for dialing down heightened emotional states. This first reinforces positive techniques for resourcing, while the latter accentuates the therapeutic response.

Going into the first cycle of EMDR, I was guided to tune in to the specific thoughts and sensations associated with the traumatic event as a point of focus. I was also asked to offer a statement about the trauma with words describing the feelings that arose. Upon recalling the trauma, I rated my level of distress, noted its presence as a tightness in my chest, and articulated my grief surrounding the trauma. Two cycles of EMDR later, the chest tightness that I associated with the lingering grief was gone.

That provided some relief, but I still needed another three cycles to calm the lingering static that I then felt in my head once the chest tightness abated. In retrospect, I believe this sensation was a somatic manifestation of self-condemnation for my role in the trauma. Blessedly, that sensation also waned after the last cycle of EMDR. With Deb's encouragement, I was guided to offer a revised statement. That statement was one of acceptance rather than guilt, which, given the accidental nature of the trauma, allowed me to separate the memory from the emotional charge—exactly what EMDR is designed to do.

Parts Work

As we round out this chapter on thinking modalities, it is worth revisiting the therapeutic application of Parts Work that was introduced in the section on subpersonalities in Chapter 5.

The most prevalent approach to Parts Work is Internal Family Systems (IFS). With IFS, different aspects of the human psyche are assigned roles, like members of a family. For example, socially awkward or repressed parts that respond with anger at being abused are called "exiled" parts, while "protector" parts have adapted to garner the approval and support of others.

The orchestrator of all these parts is referred to as "Self" by creator Richard Schwartz, and as you may recall from Chapter 5, I equate this notion with the TCM concept of the Heart-mind of the shen.

The key insight of Schwartz's work is to recognize that there are no bad parts. Although the unitary brain can shatter from trauma, as with dissociative identity disorder, multiple parts of the psyche are a natural feature in the system.

These parts may be difficult aspects of our personality that express themselves when under duress. Anger and rage may surface when one is threatened, or disgust to mask inner judgement. The IFS "Self" sees them all and knows from a clear place that each of these parts is preserving balance in the wake of trauma.

Schwartz considers the "Self" to be the undamaged essence always present and accessible behind the often louder voices of protective parts. When called upon, it can take the reins, reorganize the disparate parts, and encourage communication and understanding between them. Can we get that angry, protective part to admit it was doing the best it could and that the trauma perpetrated upon the helpless child forced a protector part to arise? The higher "Self" knows this, forgives it, and approaches protective parts with compassion and curiosity. The dialogue that ensues, guided by a psychotherapist skilled in IFS, aims to release the stigma that these parts are maladaptive.

I would broaden this understanding to include all symptoms experienced within the subconscious aspects of the body-mind. Because the subconscious doesn't speak English or any other human language, needs are communicated subtly via dreams replete with symbols or assertively via symptoms. If pain is a message that something is amiss, it is our job to translate that experience into something actionable.

Research into the efficacy of IFS for PTSD is underway. In 2021, the first funded, independently administered pilot study on this subject was accepted for publication in the *Journal of Aggression, Maltreatment & Trauma*. The study considered a constellation of symptoms characteristic of PTSD, including depression, dissociation, somatization, etc. Although the trial was not controlled, the analysis showed a significant decrease in symptoms of PTSD, bolstering the observations of decades of positive clinical outcomes witnessed by IFS therapists. Hopefully, this study will pave the way for further research.[11]

IFS looks at the culture of our psyche and elevates its purpose. With what Schwarz refers to as our "Self" in the driver's seat, we can stop wheeling around aimlessly and move forward down a path of greater awareness. Is this not a potential gift of disease? What if we stop viewing cancer as something other than ourselves and recognize it as a "part" here to teach us valuable lessons on how to live a healthy, harmonious life?

Parts Work is an exemplary psychotherapeutic approach toward wholeness directed by Heart-mind awareness. Next we turn to meditative and contemplative approaches that further define what it means to become embodied within the superconscious spiritual awareness of the energetic Heart.

10

MEDITATING THROUGH TRAUMA

"When the mind is ill at ease, the body suffers."

—Ovid, first century BCE

Hypnosis

If psychotherapy works with conscious awareness and therapies such as meridian tapping bring in an element of subconscious awareness, it raises the question whether any modality accesses superconscious awareness, what TCM describes as the shen, the spiritual awareness of the energetic Heart.

Assuredly, heart-focused meditative practices touch that aspect of human consciousness with dedicated practice. We'll explore several such modalities later in this chapter, but first, it is worth mentioning hypnotherapy as a bridge to superconscious awareness.

Consider what we've learned about psychotherapy through meridian tapping. Its efficacy speaks to the traditional-medicine notion that an energy body permeates and animates the physical body, and tapping (literally in this case) over areas of the physical body modulates the expression of the energy body. Now scale that effect to the neurological-rich nature of the heart, and a window into superconscious experience opens to insight and inspiration.

In modern biomedical parlance, the primacy of the heart as a seat of consciousness is known as energy-cardiology or cardio-energetics. The fascinating history of this area of study is detailed in *The Heart's Code: Tapping the Wisdom and Power of Our Heart Energy* by Paul Pearsall, PhD.

Pearsall writes from experience. After several persistent physical symptoms were dismissed as work stress when medical testing came back normal, he continued to experience an "impending doom" in his heart. He finally convinced his primary doctor to look deeper, and imaging revealed a tumor the size of a soccer ball in Pearsall's hip that was later diagnosed as stage 4 lymphoma.

What is most striking about Pearsall's story is how he thought about his diagnosis, even as he was going through conventional oncology treatment. By his own admission, "My cancer seemed to be the result of cells that had become heartless."

Pearsall spent much of his career studying heart intelligence and drew an interesting parallel to hypnotherapy. The neo-disassociation theory describes how hypnosis bypasses the objection of conscious awareness, while the heart, as a hidden observer, remains ever vigilant. Even as the brain yields to hypnotic suggestions such as not perceiving pain, the content of the experience can later be recalled after coming out of a hypnotic trance.

Although this does not prove conscious awareness outside of the brain and within the energetic aspect of the heart, I will remind the reader that neuroscience still debates whether consciousness resides in the body at all.

The cardio-energetic model is further strengthened by case studies of heart-transplant patients experiencing behavioral changes, cravings, and even memories that are later identified as coming from the heart donor. Such cases have been documented over the years with different organ transplants, but they predominate in heart-transplant patients. Even if only one of these cases was verified, it should be enough to open our minds to the notion of cellular consciousness.

Does hypnosis knock out the conscious objection of brain awareness and invite superconscious awareness of the heart to participate in the healing process? We next delve into the modalities of meditation, neurofeedback, and the research of the HeartMath Institute to answer this question.

Meditation and Neurofeedback

Meditation can be defined as a practice that calms the survival mind and opens the Heart-mind. Contemporary practices focus on either quieting mind chatter or letting thoughts flow freely without judgment or attachment. The former technique can be a tough slog but produces profound moments of peace and spiritual, heart-centered awareness when an elevated state is achieved. What is more often taught is the practice of letting thoughts wander while gently bringing one's attention to the breath or a point of focus, such as a candle flame.

In my book *Cancer, Stress & Mindset*, the strategy of brain-wave entrainment is discussed as a technological practice "akin to cheating while meditating." Of course, all is fair in love, war, and meditation—if listening to binaural beats can biohack the brain into a relaxed alpha or theta wave state in a fraction of the time, then its use should be promoted.

The same is true for the science surrounding neurofeedback. Originally called biofeedback, behavioral scientists in the 1960s studied methods to measure unconscious physiological processes to make them observable through a visual or auditory cue. With time, test subjects could slow their heart rate, steady breathing, relax muscles, and regulate body temperature—all signs of reducing arousal and becoming more relaxed.

Wearable devices are a modern form of neurofeedback that monitor heart rate variability (HRV) as a metric of stress resilience by quantifying the adaptability of the autonomic nervous system (ANS). If we accept the premise that PTSD is characterized by a dysregulated ANS, as shown in research literature, then HRV is one accessible method to reveal the breadth of that dysregulation and offer a means to guide the body-mind back to parasympathetic nervous system dominance.[1]

HRV is an effective strategy for inducing relaxation, but of more relevance to addressing trauma are neurofeedback devices that use electroencephalogram technology to allow the visualization of brainwave states. Here, the science supports the use of neurofeedback as an intervention for conditions such as PTSD, which disrupt cognitive function and are marked by hyperarousal.[2,3,4]

Neurofeedback has been shown to exhibit a very specific neurological effect that positions it as a notable strategy to reverse the damage done to the brain from trauma. Chronic stress and traumatic events sensitize the brain to be increasingly reactive to threat, potentially enlarging the amygdala. The anterior cingulate cortex (ACC) is an area of the brain that calms the arousal of the amygdala, and functional MRI (fMRI) studies beautifully showcase the ability of neurofeedback to normalize this relationship between the ACC and the amygdala.

Similar to neurofeedback and brainwave entrainment, meditation induces alpha brainwave states by regulating the function of the prefrontal cortex (PFC) and the ACC.[5] MRI studies at the University of Pittsburgh indicate that practicing mindfulness can decrease the gray matter volume of the amygdala and increase the volume of the PFC.[6]

All signs point to the fact that these strategies work toward building greater coherence and resilience in the nervous system, and that has broad implications for integrative cancer care. Research suggests that meditation can positively bolster the immune system. Mindfulness meditation has been shown to increase activity in the left PFC of the brain and augment immune activation.[7]

This pattern keeps repeating itself. Trauma downregulates areas of the brain involved in executive function and blunts the immune response. Practices like meditation and neurofeedback strengthen coherent activity in the brain and strengthen immunity. Not only are these statements increasingly evidenced-based, they are also patently obvious, even with nontraumatic stressful periods. College students are well aware of the letdown effect—pushing through finals week only to succumb to a head cold that sets in during a break.

If stress can so obviously blunt immunity, that suggests traumatic events can have a pronounced effect on the connection between the workings of the brain and the function of the immune system, the area of research known as psychoneuroimmunology.

That's a lot of interesting research in neuroscience, but we have gotten away from the idea that the superconscious awareness of the Heart is the ultimate destination to heal trauma and realize a return to wholeness. For clarity on that principle, we turn to the concept of coherence promoted by the HeartMath Institute.

Heart Rate Variability

Research on HRV was the mainstream offering of the HeartMath Institute but it was accompanied by a profound paradigm shift for many who practice its techniques. While meditation, brainwave entrainment, and neurofeedback can tap into superconscious awareness, the HeartMath Institute introduced a technique that is deliberate in its intent to access heart-centered consciousness. Heart-focused breathing has become the institute's foundational practice to imbue a state referred to as coherence.[8]

According to the Institute's director, Rollin McCraty, PhD, "Coherence is the state when the heart, mind, and emotions are in energetic alignment and cooperation." The subtlety of this statement requires some explanation.

The heart organ is highly neurologic, largely operating on its own, with several nerve conducting nodes that ensure the regular contractility of cardiac muscle. This is how thoracic surgeons can transplant a donor heart into a recipient and have the transplanted heart start beating again in moments. The surgical team connects vasculature but cannot rewire the heart to the patient's brain.

Whereas the nervous system of the heart takes cues from the central nervous system of the brain and spinal cord, more neurological information leaves the heart and goes to the brain than the other way around.[9] If the TCM conception of the Heart as the seat of superconscious awareness were given a voice, I'm pretty sure it would say, "I'm running the show here, thank you very much."

This is the key point behind McCraty's statement and the efficacy of the HearthMath's coherence-building techniques. HRV is an important metric of coherence, but it is a proxy for what I believe is the ultimate goal of heart-focused breathing—to restore the primacy of the energetic Heart.

Naturally, the focus of the technique is over the anatomical heart, both visualizing and feeling one's inhalation and exhalation going through the center of the chest as if the energetic Heart is pulling energy in and out with respiration. With each five- or six-second inhale, energy flows into the heart center from the front and back of the body; with each five- or six-second exhale, energy flows back outward. This is the meditative aspect of the technique.

After establishing a rhythm of breathing and keeping the focus on the heart center, the practitioner invokes a positive emotional state like care or appreciation. If you're actively stressed when starting this technique, it may take a few moments to find a positive emotion. One method is to recall a calm or happy memory and then feel what it would be like to return to that time and place. The key is to feel that emotion rather than just think about it. It is the combination of positive emotions and a focus on the heart center that generates the strongest coherence.

Practicing this technique while connected to an HRV monitor provides feedback on the quality of the state achieved. With time, it becomes easier to access and maintain coherence, building resilience and allowing increased periods of heart-centered awareness even when not connected to an HRV monitor.

Research has demonstrated that building resilience through HRV training can reduce post-deployment PTSD in military personnel when practiced as a pre-deployment strategy.[10]

To learn more about heart-focused breathing, visit the website for the HeartMath Institute or read *The HeartMath Solution: The Institute of HeartMath's Revolutionary Program for Engaging the Power of the Heart's Intelligence.*

Float Tanks

I'd like to close this chapter with a fascinating therapy that will surely see increased popularity in the coming years. Float tanks are people-sized pods filled with enough salt (usually magnesium sulfate) so that a person can effortlessly float in a closed pool of water. These tanks are designed in such a way that light and sound do not enter, and the water is heated to body temperature so that once someone has settled into an effortless buoyancy, the line between the body and the water blurs.

Another name for these pods is "sensory-deprivation tanks," but that is not an accurate description of what occurs once inside. Although sensory stimuli are reduced, the ability to feel what is happening within the body-mind is heightened. Thus, the preference for the name float tank to describe this modality.

Relaxation is the main selling point for a float tank session, with research showing a range of benefits, including decreased blood pressure, heart rate, and cortisol levels.[11] Now research has emerged using neuroimaging to study how the brain responds to a float session. One study used fMRI before and after a ninety-minute float session compared with controls sitting in a zero-gravity chair for an equivalent amount of time. Both cohorts had a reduction in "resting-state functional connectivity" within the default mode network (DMN), but the float tank group showed a more robust response.[12]

The ability to regulate the DMN may be the holy grail of stress research. In layman's terms, the DMN is the area of the brain that coordinates all the impulses that give rise to the "self" experience. One aspect of the DMN is the medial prefrontal cortex. Anything that therapeutically accesses this area can help to reframe stress and trauma.

Because they are a passive intervention, I don't consider float tanks to be a first line of therapy for deep-seated trauma, but they are a compelling resilience-building strategy. Think of it this way: If the gastrointestinal system is in turmoil, the most effective strategy is to fast. Abstaining from all food allows for a sufficient amount of rest and repair. Float tanks are a sure option to give the nervous system a fast.

I'm a big proponent of meditation, but getting into a meditative state amidst a distracting array of sights and sounds takes practice. A float tank greatly reduces these stimuli. If you are not well rested, as your nervous system unwinds, you might fall asleep while floating in a tank of salty water. But if you are alert and aware, a float tank can be an incredibly liberating somatic experience.

Not being a patentable pharmaceutical intervention, float tanks will not receive the robust research they deserve. My advice is that if there is a float-tank facility near you, try it to see if it can enhance other resilience-building strategies you are practicing.

11

MOVING THROUGH TRAUMA

"The vital force is not enclosed in man, but radiates around him like a luminous sphere, and it may be made to act at a distance. In those semi-material rays the imagination of a man may produce healthy or morbid effects."

—Paracelsus, sixteenth century CE

Energy Medicine

As a lifelong student of TCM, my career is suffused with the wisdom that a subtle energy animates the body. We call it "qi," and it is a life force that can be strengthened if weak or moved if blocked.

Living and working with qi is so ingrained into my worldview that it permeates my everyday thinking, and I have become sensitive to feeling the flow of qi in patients when performing acupuncture. Some may dismiss this notion as new age nonsense, but research into the human biofield tells a different tale.

Modern medicine is the story of the triumph of biochemistry. But before the dominance of Western pharmacology (and even herbal medicine) is a paradigm of healing based upon physics. That we are electromagnetic beings is self-evident, and thus the gentle influencing of physiology by something as simple as laying on of hands is as basic and intuitive to life as breathing. It's the gentle touch of a mother's hand on the forehead of her distressed child or the deep and heartfelt hug to soften a friend's grief.

The human biofield eluded scientific scrutiny until researchers developed sensitive enough tools to measure weak electromagnetic fields that emanate from the body. This launched the field of bioelectronics, which led to such innovations as the electrocardiogram (EKG) and MRI.

According to biophysics researcher Beverly Rubik, PhD, the human biofield is defined as "the endogenous, complex dynamic electromagnetic (EM) field resulting from the superposition of component EM fields of the organism that is proposed to be involved in self-organization and bioregulation of the organism. The components of the biofield are the EM fields contributed by each individual oscillator or electrically charged, moving particle or ensemble of particles of the organism (ion, molecule, cell, tissue, etc.), according to principles of conventional physics."[1]

Several lines of evidence support bioenergetics as an emerging field, but that research is developing and does not explain how a practice like acupuncture predates the field of biophysics by thousands of years. One explanation for the systematization of an ancient energy medicine is to consider that a small percentage of the population can actually see and feel energy around living things as colors, textures, and shapes.

This isn't that far-fetched a claim. Consider that the condition of synesthesia, the neurological cross wiring of sensory input, enables those individuals to see music and associate shapes and colors with abstract concepts like numbers and words.

To disprove the claim that all crows are black, we need only find one white crow in nature, and although albinism is rare, it exists. For seeing, feeling, and moving energy as a form of medicine, I have had the honor and privilege of studying with one such white crow.

Author of the book *Energy Medicine: Balancing Your Body's Energies for Optimal Health, Joy, and Vitality*, Donna Eden was born with the ability to see the human biofield with stunning clarity. She claims babies can see auras of energy around living beings, but few children retain that ability because of a lack of validation from non-energy-seeing adults. Whether by nurture or nature, Eden can visualize every aspect of subtle anatomy and has shared her gift by teaching thousands of people how to practice energy medicine.

There are a few aspects of energy medicine that are game

changers for healing trauma in the body. The first involves an energy system from India's traditional form of medicine, Ayurveda. Although the mapping of energetic pathways is common to both Ayurveda and TCM, the Indian system places increased emphasis on energy centers called chakras that are mainly situated along the midline of the body. Chakras are often described as spinning wheels of transformative energy, roughly corresponding to nerve plexuses or endocrine organs. When healthy, they spin in a certain direction but can rotate backward or be sluggish in their movement when affected by trauma.

For example, one such charka occupies a position in the lower pelvis. Within the precepts of energy medicine, a history of sexual trauma can be stored and perpetually affect the function of the charka in the pelvic region and/or elsewhere, such as the chakra over the heart. How a trauma is "metabolized" (or lack thereof) determines what chakras, and by extension regions, of the body will be most affected.

One technique to work through trauma is to identify the region involved, usually by the hands of a skilled energy medicine practitioner who can point out which chakras are not moving optimally. This type of energy work is often done off the body and with minimal physical contact.

Following such a consultation, the client may be given homework to "flush" the chakra by moving one's hand counterclockwise over the affected charka for a few minutes before switching to a clockwise motion to strengthen the energy center.

An even more basic technique I coach patients to try is lying relaxed and simply placing one or both hands on an area of concern while breathing deep and visualizing healthy energy pervading that space. Such a method of energy medicine is as old as the hills and takes little more than willingness and imagination. I spent many a night lying awake in bed with my hands on my belly, willing my malignant lymph nodes to heal with a silent prayer.

A technique that Eden shares is the placement of a hand over the forehead to bring energy to a pair of acupuncture points that she calls the "Oh my God!" points. They get their name from the involuntary response to experiencing shock. One might place a hand over on the forehead and utter "Oh my God!" when something unsettling occurs.

Holding a hand over the forehead leverages the warmth and energy of the hand to bring blood back to the prefrontal lobes of the brain during acute stress. Recall that the limbic system registers stress and trauma much more quickly for the sake of survival. Placing a hand on the forehead asks the brain to short-circuit the panic response and reclaim rational thinking.

Does that sound too good to be true? Next time you are inadvertently triggered, try it, and notice how much faster you return to the slower breathing and heart rate that indicate the return of parasympathetic nervous system dominance. It might take a few minutes, but keep a hand on the forehead and favor the left side.

Ongoing research in brain imaging has demonstrated a distinction between the left and right frontal lobes in processing emotions.

This was studied both as a feature of disease, with brain lesions correlating with certain emotional states, and conditions such as depression. Moreover, clinical benefit was seen with treatment of specific areas of the scalp through transcranial magnetic stimulation.[2] The evidence suggests positive emotions are most strongly associated with activity in the left prefrontal cortex, while negative emotions are more readily visualized in the right prefrontal cortex.[3]

Research documenting this effect in prefrontal asymmetry calculates it as a ratio between "right-to-left activation," and interestingly, study of an advanced mindfulness meditator showed an imbalanced ratio heavily in favor of the left prefrontal cortex, suggesting an increased propensity for positive emotions in practitioners of meditation.[4]

The implications of this research highlight the findings of intuitive practitioners of energy medicine. One interpretation is that holding a hand over the left forehead is the primary driver for the calming response elicited by the energy medicine technique. Or perhaps a harmony needs to be achieved whereby both the left and right hand play a role in restoring blood flow throughout the neocortex in opposition to the hyperarousal of the amygdala.

Whatever the case may be, it is unnecessary to own a device for transcranial magnetic stimulation of the brain. If you employ the right techniques, your hands can perform amazing feats of healing. To learn more and become better acquainted with the healthy flow of the human biofield, connect with a practitioner of Eden energy medicine.

Qigong

Many are familiar with the beautiful, flowing forms of tai chi, but the precursor practice that originated in ancient China is called qigong, which roughly translates as "energy cultivation." TCM posits that qi can be cultivated, strengthened, and moved throughout the body. Likewise, disease develops because of a deficiency or stagnation of qi. As a self-care practice, qigong is perhaps the oldest internal exercise to restore balance to the body-mind.

There are hundreds of different qigong forms that combine movements, sometimes coordinated with breathing, as well as standing and sitting meditations. My first experience with qigong was a standing posture called "holding the ball" or "hugging a tree" as the beginning warm-up for a tai chi class I attended in the back of a Chinese restaurant in the city where I grew up. I was 13 at the time, and didn't know what I was getting into. It is hard to stand with knees bent and arms rounded out in front of you while having the racing thoughts of a teenager.

Like all somatic practices, tai chi and qigong share the common thread of becoming aware of body sensations. The notion that an insubstantial force called qi animates the body is a difficult concept for cerebral westerners, but having practiced some form of qigong on and off for the last few decades, I can assure you that the ability to cultivate and circulate this vital energy is not a matter of belief. Qigong, like acupuncture, does not require one to believe in it for an effect to be realized, as evidenced by the successful veterinary application of both modalities.

Consider that guided imagery and visualization leverage thoughts to create a positive experience, but thoughts can also create a feeling of movement in the body. There is a saying in TCM that "qi flows where the mind goes," and using thoughts to generate sensations is the first step in becoming in tune with this vital energy. Here's a simple exercise to give you an idea of the power of qigong and how it can direct healing energy:

- Gently and slowly slide your finger down the inside of the opposite bare forearm from elbow to wrist. Do this several times while observing what you are doing.
- Continue this movement several more times, this time with your eyes closed.
- Now gradually lighten the pressure with each pass until you are barely touching the skin. Can you use your mind not to see but to feel that same sensation, even without direct contact?
- After noticing what you feel, open your eyes, touch the skin, and repeat the downstroke gently and slowly on the inside of the forearm.
- This time, keep your eyes open, and gradually lift off, using your intention to feel the same sensation on the skin.

Were you able to feel a sensation even without touching? Was it easier with your eyes open than closed? If you couldn't feel much, try it several days in a row to see if you can train the specific aspect of the nervous system, called proprioception, to generate a sensation with intention alone.

If you can feel movement in the body and consciously influence it, you've unlocked a universe of new possibilities. This goes beyond thinking and enters the realm of feeling change in the body. If you are stressed and your blood pressure is rising, you can feel a sinking sensation in the plumb line middle of the body (called the central channel in TCM) and, with practice, experience a significant decrease in heart rate and blood pressure.

If anxiety is rising within, ground those emotions downward by feeling roots anchor you to the floor, or better yet, deep into the earth if outside. "Breathe through your heels" is an old Taoist saying. It's not a literal phrase as your lungs stop at the diaphragm but rather a reminder to feel each inhalation extend through every aspect of your being.

This is the secret of qigong. It's not about fancy forms or mind-numbing stillness or repetitive movements. It's awareness of the movement within. With time, you can learn to feel qi as a tangible force, first between your hands and then flowing in and around the body. When I first experienced qi between my hands, it felt like pushing the same poles of two magnets together; the pushback felt tangible. That's magnetism, and with an awareness that we are electromagnetic beings, you too will feel the human biofield as an aspect of subtle anatomy that we all share.

Millions of Chinese people practice qigong daily for healing, with many visiting qigong hospitals to learn specific forms that address their disease. The most famous such hospital for cancer patients is the Zhi Neng Gong Hospital, founded in 1987 in Shijia-zhuang, Hebei, by Pang Heming, a doctor of both Western and Eastern medicine.

The name of the hospital reflects the qigong form taught, which translates "wisdom and power qigong." Pang's interest led him to work with patients with terminal cancer, and he designed a holistic health program to treat the disease.

Practitioners of qigong will be familiar with the concept of strengthening and redirecting the flow of qi in the body. Pang's methods cultivate qi for healing by accessing the storehouse of qi from nature. Many qigong students agree with this sentiment and practice outdoors, where fresh air and sunshine palpably augment the experience.

In an interview on qigong practice for healing, Pang says something very interesting that speaks to the thesis of this book— that trauma alters consciousness and healing from trauma is nothing less than a spiritual imperative:

Cultivating qi is not the most fundamental; cultivating one's spirit is. Mastery of qi is really achieved through mastery of consciousness. We use consciousness in a careful, craftsman-like way, to shape our life, to attain our goals. If we use modern terminology to name this process, we call it qigong. The ancients used the word qi and this mystifies people. But in modern terms, qigong is just a refinement of consciousness to enhance the state of qi in the body. This leads to vibrant health, a harmonious body and mind, and an awakened spiritual life.[5]

Many of the cancer patients that arrived at Zhi Neng Gong Hospital seeking a cure for their disease were given a prognosis of only months left to live. Pang was clear in the interview that their cure rate is very low, at about 5%, yet documenting the cure of even a single terminal patient should open our eyes to what might be possible with what he calls "an awakened spiritual life". In his own words:

Our cancer patients, even though they die, don't suffer greatly. They don't need medicines and anesthetics. They're not emaciated or dispirited when they die. Some patients arrive as thin as a ghost. After practice, they put on weight. Some die almost a pleasant death while asleep. Others died while on the practice field—they take a break and die. Two died that way recently. We can say they died with real dignity.[6]

In the western world where the fear surrounding oncology treatment and a slow, horrific decline is compounded on top of the threat of the disease itself, it is a gift to realize an awakened spiritual life amidst all adversity. It makes me appreciate how addressing trauma and the realization of one's quintessential spiritual nature are the essence of all healing. While a cancer cure may not be possible, healing is always available to us.

Somatic Experiencing®

The work of Peter Levine, PhD, focuses on a somatic approach to healing trauma. The broader field is called sensorimotor psychotherapy, but Levine promoted the term "Somatic Experiencing" (SE), implying the therapy's ability to help heal the past by guiding the participant to become more body aware in the present.

One of the central themes in trauma research is that an unresolved freeze response predisposes disassociation. The resultant disconnect in body awareness often leads to an inability to describe one's emotions, called alexithymia in psychiatry. Thus, the aim of somatic therapy is to reinstate a body-centered awareness. Before delving in to how SE accomplishes this, a quick review of the nervous system is in order. Acute stress activates the sympathetic nervous system to respond via "fight" or "flight." Whether running toward a threat or away from it, the response is action.

A third response is one that Levine highlights as a common reaction to severe trauma—dissociation. The activation of the dorsal vagal complex is thought to be the oldest evolutionary response to life-threatening circumstances and is common among mammals and reptiles. When threatened, they freeze and play dead. This may dissuade a predator from completing the kill of the prey animal, or if the predator does resume the hunt, the altered state of dissociation may grant to the prey animal an inability to feel pain prior to its demise.

With humans, the freeze response has a broader implication. In Levine's own words from his seminal work *Waking the Tiger: Healing Trauma*, "Posttraumatic symptoms are, fundamentally, incomplete physiological responses suspended in fear." By this, Levine implies that trauma results from an instinctual cycle that is overridden by our neocortex and rendered incomplete. Dissociation is a strong predictor of developing PTSD, and humans tend not to shake off trauma, both metaphorically and literally, as easily as other animals.

Levine provides an interesting observation of nature that imbues hope for a body-focused strategy to resolve trauma. A hallmark of SE is to release (or discharge) the energy of dissociation that comes from the freeze response. Animals do this by shivering or shaking following a traumatic event. And it's not a slight tremor; we're talking about a full body trembling that goes on as long as necessary until the nervous system rebalances itself.

Humans do this too. I can think of several occurrences of seeing children who endure a close call (of something that could have been disastrous—such as a fall from a height), immediately start shaking when comprehension of the consequences of their actions sets in. That existential fear gets shaken off with high efficiency. Sometimes, when adults experience trauma, they respond with shaking; at other times, they suppress this innate response.

Perhaps we deem trembling a sign of weakness or unbecoming in a social situation? Whatever the reason humans deny their instincts, the observation by Levine in the framework of SE is that the release of pent-up and frozen energy from trauma results in involuntary trembling.

Tingling, heat, and a generalized feeling of movement in the body are also signs of an awareness and releasing of an area affected by trauma. What matters, according to Levine, is that our response to a threatening event is more important than the event that caused it. Thus, we can access the feelings frozen within us without replaying the trauma and risk reliving the event, completing the cycle of healing.

Our awareness of body sensations is accomplished by a deep listening and responding to what Levine refers to as our "felt sense," a term coined in the 1950s by Eugene Gendlin, a student of Carl Rogers, of the humanistic psychology tradition. The ability to articulate sensations is the heart of working with felt sense.

The technical term for internal awareness is interoception, but the notion of felt sense goes beyond just a basic awareness of physiological processes. Most people can tune in to their breathing or heartbeats. Feeling where grief is stuck in the body is a different perceptual skill but one that can be cultivated. Felt sense is the domain of subconscious awareness, and intuition is the language it speaks.

Levine's hallmarks of a traumatic reaction include hyper-arousal, constriction, dissociation, and freezing (immobility). The somatic symptoms these components produce are identified through felt sense and connected to an incomplete survival response. "Digestive issues, especially irritable bowel syndrome, chronic fatigue, asthma, joint and muscle pain, chronic regional pain (fibromyalgia), and migraines are all examples of symptoms that can be somatic in origin," writes the late PTSD researcher Joseph A. Boscarino, PhD, in his lauded paper on the subject, "Posttraumatic Stress Disorder and Physical Illness: Results from Clinical and Epidemiologic Studies."

Consider how this might apply to a cancer patient: few are strong enough to withstand the dissociation that results from being diagnosed with cancer. Let's assume that a compassionate health care team swoops in to address the illness, and remission is achieved. Thereafter, little attention is given to the emotional stability of the patient in the months and years that follow. For many of us, not a day goes by that we don't think about cancer. For the less fortunate among us, we live with an ongoing fear of relapse.

In the trauma literature, there is an acknowledged phenomenon of reenactment. People who have been traumatized are drawn to situations that recapitulate the original event. It is as if the body is trying to complete the cycle of healing and, in the absence of somatic therapy in a safe clinical setting, the body seeks the familiar, although painful, circumstances of an analogous traumatic situation. Renowned psychotherapist Sigmund Freud called this "repetition compulsion," and he posited that the reliving of trauma in relationships or the replaying of them in dreams were opportunities to learn novel solutions.

Now consider a cancer patient in remission going for follow-up visits, getting scans, and waiting for the results. These are all necessary aspects of patient management, but they are also powerful reminders of the emotional and physical trauma wrought upon the body-mind during conventional oncology treatment. I don't like to think about cancer relapse as a self-fulfilling prophecy, but all the hallmarks of an unresolved healing response are there and we would do well to acknowledge any symptoms that arise from these routine follow-up appointments. If we can all agree that "white coat syndrome" is the transient increase in blood pressure by a healthy person during a routine doctor visit, what rehashing is a cancer patient prone to when visiting an oncologist?

In terms of trauma as a cause of cancer, while a malignant tumor is not conventionally thought to have a psychosomatic origin, the importance of adopting a somatic approach to resolve trauma—and by extension, I would argue, cancer—is that symptoms stemming from dissociation are unequivocal signs of a disruption in the terrain (health) of the body. By addressing somatic symptoms, we restore agency and resilience to the body-mind. There's no downside to adopting this mindset and pursuing therapy to that end.

Holistic medical providers sometimes say patients "carry their issues in their tissues." Providers working in integrative oncology are dedicated to understanding the emotional roots of cancer. It's not a stretch for a practitioner of TCM to equate the stagnancy of emotions with the formation of a tumor. Conventional oncologists may dismiss these statements, but once we acknowledge that the body, mind, and spirit are one, it is self-evident that psychosomatic factors contribute to cancer development.

Deactivating Trauma with Somatic Experiencing

I booked a virtual visit with a friend and colleague, Katie Fritz, to learn to better access felt sense through SE. Katie integrated SE into her TCM practice as a method to reinforce embodiment.

Like so many of us in health care, Katie observed escalating stress, busyness, and the tendency to self-medicate rather than address trauma and emotional suffering. We can try to talk through those issues, but Katie was quick to point out that traumatized people are smart and may not get benefit from cognitive behavioral therapy if they choose to spin the narrative to avoid bringing up deep issues.

The solution is a return to somatic therapies because, as she puts it, "The body never lies." Katie uses SE to assess the set point of a patient's nervous system, then begins the session by establishing the groundwork for feeling safe.

For my session, this began with sitting comfortably in a chair while slowly casting my gaze around the room and taking notice of my surroundings. This gave my brain something neutral to do as I focused more on the sensations arising in my body.

Katie then coached me to track sensations and notice the areas that felt comfortable. This act of "resourcing" was the anchor before noticing other areas that felt tight or stuck. My challenged areas were the left side of my body, especially the back of my shoulder and neck. With closed eyes while tracking the sensations on the left side, I gave voice to its quality with whatever words came to mind. Katie gently affirmed my discovery but directed me deeper into the experience by questioning whether a color, texture, or word came to mind in connection with this sensation. As a word popped into my awareness, I didn't wish to utter it aloud, in part because the very word made me uncomfortable and stating it did not come without shame.

Feeling my hesitancy, Katie quickly affirmed that I need not share the word aloud, but I did and was glad for it. The moment I confessed the emotion linked to the sensation on the left side of my body, a rush of prickly heat surfaced. Seeing the visible manifestation of my activation, Katie talked me through the pendulation process, shifting my focus to the feel-good right side of my body and carrying that sensation to the left side.

After a few minutes of pendulation, the heat dissipated, and the left side of my body now felt as pleasantly relaxed as the right side. This completed one cycle of activation and deactivation—the culmination of one session of SE.

The final step was to open my eyes and again gaze slowly around the room. Aside from anchoring the session at its close, I noted how freely I turned my head to the left to take in my surroundings, where before I only briefly looked left before focusing the majority of my attention off to the right side.

This may seem like a minor detail, but it reflected a relative favoring of my right side that was now more balanced. It was at this moment that I recalled my history with Bell's palsy over a decade earlier. The left-sided facial paralysis was accompanied by an intense pain in the left ear and back of the neck.

While I've largely healed from that malady, I still have a minor amount of residual nerve damage. Perhaps remnants of that trauma surfaced because of my attention to the sensation and the associated word?

Overall, the experience was quite liberating, and it granted me a greater appreciation for becoming more body aware. I now understand how the practice of SE can safely release the pent-up energy of past traumas.

I asked Katie if this was a practice one could do on one's own, akin to meditation. Her answer was as pertinent as it was wise. She offered that we've all experienced some degree of relational trauma and that there is a benefit to working with a compassionate practitioner. This helps repair trust in relationships that may have been damaged in challenging past encounters.

Arts and Movement

"The body keeps the score, and movement is medicine."

—Bessel van der Kolk. MD

With an increased academic focus on science, technology, engineering, and math has come a decrease in children being exposed to the arts. The result may very well be multiple generations of adults who are good at thinking and lackluster in expressing themselves. Balancing intelligence quotient with emotional quotient is essential to being well rounded.

The arts have their greatest value in making life worth living, and their healing potential is vast. Among the different types of art therapy, there are a few that are highly scalable, such as painting, sculpting, theater, music, and dance.

Trauma-informed theater has successfully been implemented in New York City, where The Possibility Project is helping area youth resolve conflict through nonviolent means. The project's website says, "Our young people commit to meeting for six to seven hours weekly over the course of nine months to engage in a social/emotional learning experience that uses the performing arts to examine and address the personal and social forces that shape their lives and identities."

Music is another area of the arts that transforms our experience. There is a reason blues music exists and that musicians expressing sadness and grief prefer songs in minor keys. Melody and rhythm allow us to feel different emotions that change depending on the style of music. Marches motivate, while lullabies soothe. Violin strings can pull on our heart strings, while a chorus of human voices in a cathedral can make one's entire body buzz.

If these experiences are unfamiliar to you, I would encourage a simple exercise. Attend a drum circle where you're provided with a drum to play, and experience your body reacting to a group of individuals in sync with the same rhythm.

The first time I joined a drum circle, I was surprised at how natural it felt. Even though I never thought of myself as musically inclined, I've learned that almost anyone can drum. If you let it in, the steady rhythm of several drummers creates space for deep emotional expression.

A 2008 study in the journal *The Arts in Psychotherapy* explored just that effect. Veterans who suffered from combat-induced PTSD saw a reduction in their PTSD symptoms following a drumming session. This included "non-intimidating access to traumatic memories," an effect even more powerful when you consider that group drumming among PTSD sufferers allowed for increased feelings of openness and togetherness with other traumatized veterans.[7]

Finally, consider dance and other forms of guided movement, such as eurythmy and tai chi. As we've already established from therapies like EMDR, trauma impairs the brain's inability to process bilaterally. The simple act of walking, where the right arm swings in counterpoint to the left leg (and vice versa) is an exercise in getting the body's energy to cross over. Movement therapies provide consistent bilateral, rhythmic stimulation.

Yoga is a form of movement that has been clinically researched for its stress-reducing effects. More relevant to this work is a spin-off modality called trauma-informed yoga, practiced as an embodied intervention for healing PTSD.

A 2014 paper supported by the National Institutes of Health found that a ten-week intervention of weekly trauma-informed yoga provided significant benefit to treat PTSD, with "effect sizes comparable to well-researched psychotherapeutic and psychopharmacologic approaches." The study concluded that yoga "may improve the function of traumatized individuals by helping them to tolerate physical and sensory experiences associated with fear and helplessness and to increase emotional awareness and affect tolerance."[8]

The Purple Dot Yoga Project has been the leading resource for trauma-informed yoga programs and teacher training. According to the project's website, "When we gain access and autonomy over our physical bodies—through movement and mindfulness practice—we create space to unravel painful and traumatic memories that are stored in our bodies and locked deep in our nervous system and minds."

Dance therapy has been studied among African adolescent survivors of war. Implemented alongside group psychotherapy, improvisational dancing allowed former teenage soldiers to "demonstrate their wartime experiences through public presentation of a role-play."[9]

This last study demonstrates an important point: results are stronger when combining modalities, such as free dancing to the entraining rhythm of a drum. Picturing our indigenous ancestors dancing around a fire to the beat of drums suddenly feels less like a party and more like group therapy. How amazing that these expressions of sound and movement can be as much a healing ritual as a celebration of life. Clearly, we have lost much wisdom becoming "civilized." If trauma is characterized by the freeze response, moving through it with theater, music, dance, and yoga are subtle but powerful ways to becoming unstuck without rehashing past events.

Breath Work

Whether practicing yoga, performing theater, or being guided through a somatic exercise, breath is the common movement tying together meditative and movement therapies. Being mindful of the rhythm of inhalation and exhalation is the most viscerally grounding movement experience we have access to.

Consider that a shift from normal relaxed respiration is an early sign that the nervous system has shifted from parasympathetic dominance to a state of sympathetic arousal. Breathing may become shallow and restrictive, or hyperventilation may begin the cascade of sweating and increased heart rate. Breathing lies at the intersection between calm and the stress-hormone cascade characteristic of trauma and PTSD.

Over the last several years, I have had infrequent episodes of waking in the middle of the night with a feeling of terror but no recollection of being in a nightmare. Perhaps the best way to describe it is having a panic attack while sleeping. (I've never had a panic attack while awake, so I can only speculate on that point.) I awaken with a whole-body convulsion in a cold sweat and feeling like my heart is about to explode from my chest—all accompanied by an intense free-floating anxiety.

The first time this happened, I barely slept the rest of the night and was a wreck for several days. The most recent occurrence (while writing this book) was a demonstrably different experience. Upon my convulsive awakening and feeling the panic rising, my nervous system took over, and I immediately began box breathing. For those unfamiliar with the technique, visualize a box with square proportions. The four sides represent inhalation, holding the breath, exhalation, and holding the emptiness—each for an equivalent amount of time. Each segment is typically performed in intervals of five to seven seconds.

I'd like to think that my enlightened prefrontal cortex rationalized that I was in an extreme stress response, and therefore slowing respiration with box breathing was a good idea. But instead, I fell—blessedly—to the level of my training. Every morning, following my sitting meditation, I practice several breathing exercises. The first among them is box breathing, where I breathe in, hold, breathe out, and hold for six seconds for each segment.

When confronted with my middle-of-the-night wake-up call, I began box breathing. It was difficult at first because I was mightily distracted by a feeling of dread, but I kept at it, and my heart rate normalized within a few minutes. I still had a hard time falling asleep, but I quickly blunted the stress response.

Breath control is even more powerful if you can go one step further and stop a stress response before it is elicited. Sometimes that's unavoidable, such as when the car driving in front of you brakes suddenly. If you know you are about to enter a stressful situation, getting your breathing right can sometimes nip the stress response in the bud. Military special forces learn box breathing, but they give it the more valiant name "tactical breathing," and teach its use when under fire (sometimes literally) during a mission.

The salient point is that breathing is the pivot point between sympathetic and parasympathetic nervous system responses. Whether or not consciously controlled, meditation and movement therapies help guide respiration toward a slow, rhythmic, and calm pattern. Practicing breath work, either as a stand-alone practice or alongside other aforementioned therapies, adds another layer of somatic unwinding and greater control over the stresses of life.

12

DREAMING THROUGH TRAUMA

"Sleep is that which most effectively and widely frees the mind from all external disturbances."

—Aristotle, fourth century BCE

Time heals all wounds, and the healing power of sleep may be why that adage exists. Those under intense emotional duress may experience nightmares but may also be blessed with deep, dissociative sleep. Peaceful dreaming may also be part of the healing response as the richness of rapid eye movement (REM) sleep communicates insight to help resolve, or at least soften, emotional upheaval.

To understand dreaming as an agent of change, it is necessary to appreciate the fluidity of consciousness during sleep. Even in the absence of acute trauma, one night may involve dreaming of being in an alien world and the next a unique consciousness divorced from any reality associated with the ego identification of "self." In a dreamscape, it is possible to be a completely different person.

Perhaps the most bizarre manifestation of how disparate the dreamworld can be from waking reality is the initial REM onset that occurs when falling asleep. As an early bird married to a night owl, I have drifted off to sleep half aware of my physical surroundings and half floating off in a dream. Easily roused during this light sleep by my wife slipping into bed, I awake to full consciousness, unable to recall the dream I was having seconds prior. Over the years, I have made more attempts than I can count to recapture the content of these dreams. My mind is simply incapable of reclaiming that dreamy state. What a mystery of consciousness!

Waking out of a deep sleep is stranger still. It can sometimes take several seconds to anchor consciousness back in the body in which "self" becomes identified with the physical. Where does consciousness go? Why do we come back as a consistent "self," and where do these other personalities reside? Some of the world's greatest philosophers and researchers have attempted to answer these questions. Any perspective we can glean is only the tip of a massive iceberg of consciousness.

Lacking concrete answers to the fluidity of consciousness need not stop us from directing dreaming toward deep emotional healing. One theory for the role of REM sleep is the consolidating of waking experience for cataloging in long-term memory.[1]

Problem solving and learning is accelerated when the waking consciousness takes a back seat to workings of the subconscious. These terms, borrowed from psychology, may not be the best fit in this context, so let's discuss sleep from the TCM paradigm.

Recall that the major organs have spiritual forces associated with them, loosely correlated with Western esoteric concepts. The Liver houses the Hun spirit, akin to the astral body. This is the aspect of consciousness that leaves the body during sleep and enters the dreamworld to process life separate from the physical and etheric (or energy) body. This dissociation is where healing occurs. The autonomic processes of the body heal under the influence of the parasympathetic nervous system. We rest, digest, and recover.

Meanwhile, the mental sphere travels with the Hun spirit and "digests" the conscious experience of waking life. This is when and where insights can flood into our being, problems can find resolution, and the damaging effects of trauma soften. It's an act of grace of the highest order.

Where consciousness goes during this time is mystifying, but it might have something to do with how we experience reality. In waking life, we organize life around three dimensions of space and one dimension of time. For example, arranging a meeting requires directions to be given on an x, y, and z axis of space, such as the third floor of the building on the corner of Fifth and Main streets. That covers the three spatial dimensions, and then stipulating a meeting time adds the fourth dimension, time.

I've often wondered if arrival into the dreamscape inverts the laws of physics such that consciousness experiences three dimensions of time and one of space. A healing dream may encompass experiencing a past emotional upset, but seeing it from a different perspective or dreaming of successfully completing a future challenge to blunt the anxiety associated with it. Many will have had the experience of preparing for a performance, such as public speaking, a sporting competition, or a musical recital, and dreamed the desired outcome.

The salient point is that time is remarkably fluid in a dream state, such that movement between past, present, and future is possible. As for space, there is no discernible x, y, or z axis in a dreamscape. Spatially, consciousness collapses to a singular focus, while we can move back and forth through time as effortlessly as navigating city streets when awake.

This inversion of dimensionality may be what enables creative thought and emotional resolution while dreaming. Healthy dissociation grants the physical and energy body a chance to heal from the onslaught of mental and emotional stress placed upon it during the waking hours, whereas the aspect of consciousness represented by the Hun spirit (or astral body) can process thoughts and emotions by experiencing them outside of time.

That's a lot of insubstantial speculation, so let's ground it into something actionable. Dreams can be a terrifying reliving of trauma, or they can support their healing. Although dreams cannot always be controlled, they can be influenced. If the emotional upset is acute, chances are, fitful dreams will be interspersed with periods of deep, nonresponsive sleep. The sleeping brain is always trying to make sense of emotionally charged experiences, parsing out what is relevant and storing it as memories.[2]

Initiating proactive, healing dreams starts with intention. Take the concerning matter at hand, and think or journal about it just before going to sleep. Hash out everything that is worrying and all the associated emotions. If you've recently been diagnosed with cancer or are experiencing symptoms suggestive of a relapse, talk or write it out. What are your fears?

Consciously air out as much of the unrest as possible to give the subconscious material to work with in a dream state. Then comes auto-suggestion, a fancy word for hypnotizing oneself. This does not require a formal induction process. Simply invite healing and resolution into your dreams in the moments before you fall asleep. You've already expressed what is concerning you; now place a hand over your heart as you rest in bed, deepen your breathing, and intend for healing to occur while asleep and dreaming.

Those of a religious disposition will immediately recognize this process as a form of prayer, imploring a higher spiritual power for guidance as the veil thins during sleep. Those with an agnostic or atheistic worldview can leverage this effect by acknowledging neuroplasticity and the evolutionary benefit of restorative sleep to imbue a survival advantage. These notions are not mutually exclusive, but choose the narrative that resonates with you; whether by creation or evolution (or both), trust your nervous system.

Sleep is an embodied reminder that conscious awareness need not micromanage healing.

The final step is acknowledging the content of dreams upon waking. Sometimes it will be obvious: a dream of reviewing a clean PET scan with your oncologist and waking with a feeling of optimism. Other times, dreams will speak in metaphors requiring translation. Dreaming of floating in a calm body of water may suggest that the stillness of meditation will best address the current predicament. Listen and adapt.

Keep a dream journal and look for patterns. This could be jotting down a few words to jog a memory of the dream. A variant of this is to view the events of the dream as a film and write a title that encapsulates it. Or a dream journal can be quite detailed, describing sounds, sights, emotions, etc. Whatever technique you choose, be sure to do it as soon as you wake up (whether in the morning or middle of the night) to capture as much of your imagery and feelings as possible. Dreams arise from a deep state of consciousness that is tenuous to recall in waking consciousness. Take advantage of the state between sleep cycles or upon rising to record the contents of dreams.

A fascinating paper in the journal *Explore* specifically delves into the possibility that dreams can portend a cancer diagnosis. Eighteen women with documented breast cancer completed a survey about health-related dreams before their diagnosis. The results claimed that "The five most common characteristics of warning dreams in descending order of frequency reported in the survey were: a sense of conviction about their importance in 94%; the dreams were more vivid, real or intense than ordinary in 83%; an emotional sense of threat, menace or dread in 72%; the use of the specific words breast cancer/tumor in 44%; and the sense of physical contact with the breast in 39%."[3]

This was a small retrospective survey without a control group, but it was followed up by a pilot study to gain clarity on the number of patients needed to provide statistical analysis for dreams being predictive of a cancer diagnosis. Data was collected via an anonymous survey of 163 women receiving a breast biopsy, with 64% of them reporting that they usually remember their dreams and only 5% keeping a dream journal. If we consider those women who do not remember their dreams as an informal control group, then of the women who recalled and/or recorded their dreams, almost 12% had dreams containing the word "cancer" before or just after their biopsy.[4]

Further research is needed to separate the signal from the noise with something as subtle as dream prognostication. Yet the potential for dream diagnosis has long been a part of ancient healing traditions ranging from those of Native Americans to the Grecian roots of modern medicine. In the temples of Asclepius, dreams were revered for their diagnostic value. The priests of the temple used the content of dreams experienced while under their care to guide treatment.[5]

As the inheritor of the Asclepian tradition, allopathic medicine has largely forsaken the predictive potential of dreams, though the cultural acknowledgment of messages from the sub-conscious mind persists in those who keep a dream journal.

We don't know how often such nighttime prognostication occurs, but its mere occurrence strengthens the argument that the wisdom of the subconscious mind is more profound than we acknowledge. This is especially true for trauma, which can be repressed beyond conscious awareness. Healing occurs on many levels while we sleep.

Generally speaking, there are two aspects to restorative sleep. Within the ninety-minute sleep cycles that occur over an average eight-hour period, deep sleep predominates in the first half of the night. This is the phase of sleep that is most regenerative to the physical body. If recovering from an injury, much of the healing will occur during this first phase.

Just past the midpoint of an eight-hour night of sleep, the focus switches from deep sleep toward dream-filled REM sleep. This is partly why it is easier to recall a dream upon waking first thing in the morning compared to within the first few hours of sleep. We dream all night long, but dreams will be longer closer to morning. REM sleep is more restorative to mental and emotional health as the brain processes experiences from the days prior and catalogs memory.

This cursory understanding of sleep cycles is important to point out as the portion of sleep that is missed during a truncated night of rest is, by default, the REM phase. If the body-mind only receives six hours of sleep when it requires eight, that could amount to upwards of 40–50% less REM sleep.

With no other intentional intervention, the brain heals the psyche from trauma by rewriting the narrative of our experience during REM periods of sleep. That might be a difficult task if recovering from severe trauma where nightmarish images are all the brain can conjure, but problem solving and emotional upset can more readily be reframed during REM sleep.

The plot thickens when you consider there are ways to "dream" while awake. We'll explore one way in the next section and another in the next chapter.

Psychedelic-Assisted Psychotherapy

Watching the documentary film *Fantastic Fungi* was as emotionally moving as it was educational. In one segment, the filmmakers take us into the treatment room at Johns Hopkins Medical Center to follow the journey of two participants taking psilocybin, the active psychotropic compound in so-called magic mushrooms. Both were cancer patients struggling with anxiety surrounding their diagnosis and mortality. Hearing them convey the existential freedom they embodied from just one guided session of psilocybin had me reaching for the tissue box.

There are many faces behind the revival of psychotropics as therapeutic tools, one recent advocate being author and journalist

Michael Pollan, who brought mainstream attention to the issue in his book and subsequent TV series, *How to Change Your Mind.* Pollan covers the transition of psilocybin and 3,4-methylenedioxy methamphetamine (MDMA) from being categorized as Schedule 1 drugs (no medical use) by the Controlled Substances Act, to phase 2 and 3 clinical trials that showcase these substances' clear therapeutic potential.

While some may cringe at the thought of taking a mind-altering substance, in a therapeutic setting, these compounds are receiving a renaissance of use in two particular realms germane to this book. The first is psilocybin being studied for end-of-life anxiety in cancer patients. The second is MDMA alongside psychotherapy to treat PTSD.

A randomized, double-blind trial that administered psilocybin to cancer patients showed a significant and sustained decrease in depression and anxiety for patients who have received a life-threatening cancer diagnosis.[6] Where before there was only despair, this powerful mycological medicine guides the patient on a journey of ego dissolution where the fear of dying gives way to peace and acceptance. I can think of nothing more healing for a body on the cusp of death than to realize the eternal nature of spirit.

MDMA saw widespread therapeutic use by psychotherapists for years before it became a recreational drug. Instead of controlling its street use in deference to the pleas of psychotherapists documenting clear medical benefit, the politics of the time forbade its use by medical professionals. Psychotherapists administered

MDMA because of its action as an empathogen, which helps a person to feel empathy. MDMA has seen a resurgence in use to help those struggling with PTSD revisit and heal from traumatic experiences without becoming re-traumatized. It softens the edges of painful memories so that conventional talk therapy can guide the patient to realize self-empathy, liberating the psyche from victim consciousness.

A longitudinal pooled analysis of six phase 2 trials of MDMA-assisted psychotherapy for PTSD showed that treatment effects were sustained for at least one year following the therapy sessions. That's incredible when you consider how brief and inexpensive the intervention is.[7]

At the time of this writing, a randomized, double-blind, placebo-controlled multisite phase 3 study of the efficacy and safety of MDMA-assisted psychotherapy for the treatment of PTSD is complete and awaiting publication.

It is only a matter of time before both psilocybin and MDMA are reclassified as viable medical interventions prescribable by psychiatrists. This is key—these substances have maximum thera-peutic potential and minimum risk when given in a professional medical setting where psychotherapists help the patient integrate the experience. Prescreening patients and clarifying their intent predisposes the best possible outcome from these powerful drugs. Context is king with psychotropics.

MDMA will certainly see broad acceptance and use for treating PTSD. Alongside psychotherapy, MDMA will surely become one of the most effective treatments for allowing the rational part of the prefrontal cortex to contextualize trauma entrenched in the limbic system of the emotional midbrain.

My hope for psilocybin is that it sees widespread use in a therapeutic setting well before cancer patients are terminal. Consider the therapeutic potential of a cancer patient being free of the fear of death at the front end of treatment instead of the back end. This shift in mindset could lead to a breakthrough in oncology treatment, helping patients realize their "why" for being and empowering adherence to treatment and lifestyle changes.

There is one other psychotropic drug worth mentioning, not only because it has therapeutic potential for treating PTSD but because it is legal, inexpensive (off patent), and widely available. Ketamine has a long history of use as an anesthetic at high doses, but at a dose below the threshold of full consciousness dissolution, the drug has a marked psychotropic effect that is favorable to a psychotherapeutic setting.[8]

In addition to spearheading research using ketamine for the treatment of PTSD in veterans, the Ketamine Research Foundation is attempting to define a new clinical diagnosis called "posttraumatic stress disorder—life threatening illness (PTSD-LTI)," most acutely applicable to cancer survivors.

Ketamine is a dissociative, but unlike the dissociation brought on by the shock of trauma, ketamine acts as an embodied dissociative, meaning it allows you to experience a cognitive reset within the body instead of being disconnected from it. This is a different pharmacological effect from the visionary effects of psilocybin or the empathic effects of MDMA.

The word "dissociation" may not best describe the mental state brought on by ketamine. Researchers have proposed other terms, like derealization or depersonalization, that emphasize the positive effects of stepping outside one's cognitive bias.

One mechanism suggested for ketamine's cognitive reset is its effect on glutamate. As the most common excitatory neurotransmitter in the brain, the modulation of glutamate receptors is speculated to underlie ketamine's potential use in treating depression.[9]

Unlike psilocybin and MDMA, ketamine has an abuse potential, not because of chemical addiction but from psychological dependance. That risk is minimized because only licensed psychiatrists in a psychotherapeutic environment can access the drug.

A network of providers practicing ketamine-assisted psychotherapy can be found on the Ketamine Psychotherapy Associates website, and telemedicine for patients with anxiety and/or depression is accessible via the online service Mindbloom.

Psychedelic-Assisted Spirituality

The combination of low-dose psychotropics with psychotherapy is poised to become a dominant healing modality for trauma. The key to this strategy is the pairing. While the former reboots the nervous system, the latter is critical for integration.

Before modern psychotherapy, shamans and medicine men and woman used psychotropic plants within indigenous cultures for thousands of years. Inherent in that context is a ritualistic ceremony occurring in nature, alongside a supportive community, and above all, acknowledgment of the spiritual dimension of life.

It is within this context that I ingested a high dose of psilocybin-containing mushrooms with the intent to explore the potential for plant medicine to awaken and deepen spiritual connection. Early one fall morning, a trusted and experienced guide and I ventured out into the woods and settled on a glade, a beautiful setting overlooking a prairie on the edge of a mature forest. My intent was that my journey be safe, meaningful, and healing.

The several-hour experience was comfortable and not unfamiliar territory because of all the inner work I've done over the years. The novel part of the journey was the conglomeration of experiences. If pressed for a description, I would describe it as feeling like deep meditation, shamanic journeying, cranio-sacral therapy, and Christmas all rolled into one.

The first hour brought on the paradoxical body heaviness and lightheadedness that required me to lie on my back and surrender to the experience. I expected this, based on a trial several months prior with a low dose of psilocybin mushroom, an experiment to prepare for this high-dose journey.

As the heaviness fully descended during the peak of the experience, my breathing slowed, and I effortlessly opened into a deep meditative state that takes me some time to achieve during my regular morning sitting meditation practice. I heard the sounds of nature around me, but the stillness and quiet were undisturbed by them.

Within the solitude of the eternal moment, the boundaries of my body blurred, and I felt respiration extend beyond my body to include the surrounding landscape. I thought at first that the ground that supported me was breathing too, but realized that the rhythm was much slower than the typical cycles of inhalation and exhalation. Having spent many hours receiving craniosacral therapy, I realized that the feeling was akin to the sensation of the therapist initiating a "still point" where you can feel the slow pulsation of cerebrospinal fluid moving. In this instance, I felt that pulsation in entrainment with the earth's own rhythm.

It is important to point out that many who ingest psychotropics experience marked visual hallucinations that showcase the synesthesia that these substances can induce. This was not the case for me, with the thrust of my experience being kinesthetic. During the peak, I felt everything going on inside me and a heightened sense of my surroundings. This is very characteristic of any peak meditation I've experienced where the focus shifts from "doing" to "being."

The visual information that I did receive was similar to how I "see" when shamanic journeying to the steady rhythm of a drum, a practice that I've frequented over the last 20 years. In that state, my mind's eye could easily visualize the one prominent symbol and message that crowned the peak experience.

As the stillness of the peak experience subsided, my emotional body opened up. I can best describe the emotion as the soft joy of Christmas—not the morning with all its excitement, but the evening once the hype has died down. It reminded me of a quiet evening, full from the Christmas feast and sitting by the fire cuddling my wife and daughter. This feeling of coziness and warmth pervaded my being; tears gently surfaced.

A few hours after ingestion, I was back on my feet, observing the natural world around me with childlike wonder as all my senses remained heightened for a time.

I did not go into this experience thinking about my history of trauma, but I came away with an important lesson regarding how we can heal from pain and suffering when embracing the spiritual dimension of life.

The night before my psychedelic journey, I was up late into the night, restless with the heaviness of several things. I had not planned it, but my trip to the woods the next morning was to be the exact one-year anniversary of my last hospitalization from a bowel obstruction. Although going a year without another such episode was progress, I felt the weight of the last several years since my cancer diagnosis.

Another matter was the acute grief and guilt from the death of a pet that occurred earlier in the month. Being an accidental death in which I played a role, images of the event still revisited my consciousness, especially in the dark of night.

The third disturbing thought came when tucking my daughter into bed. She shared that one child from our school community had been in the hospital the last month with her third bout of cancer. Even with all my contemplations on living and learning from cancer, I simply can't tolerate the thought of a child stricken with the disease. It defies my ability to be rational, and the thought of what this child's family must be going through left me feeling broken. Sometime after 1 a.m., I finally fell asleep.

This was the heaviness that walked with me through the woods to the site of my journey. On the other side of the experience, the message was clear: pain and trauma don't go away, but it is possible for those heavy feelings to coexist with the lightness of joy.

Psychotropics won't take you to the top of the mountain, but they will give you a glimpse of what is up there and, thus, what is possible if you do the work. Peak experiences can readily occur through meditation, breath work, vigorous exercise, etc. To cultivate a calm state of being is undoubtedly an arduous climb, and all our pain doesn't get left behind as we summit—the scars of life journey with us.

The joy I felt at the end of my plant-medicine journey is a reminder that emotional pain can soften with time, but even if it never goes away, there is still—always—a place for joy.

Herbal Medicine

Psychotropic drugs are not for everyone, but there are more gentle and gradual options for those struggling with the fallout from trauma. These include herbal preparations with a long history of use as calming agents.

From the botanical world, three well-loved and meticulously researched herbs are worthy of discussion. The first and most gentle is lemon balm (*Melissa officinalis*), which is both calming and restorative to the nervous system. One significant benefit to lemon balm is that it is widely available and can be easily grown in a home herb garden. Lemon balm is vigorous to the point of being potentially invasive, so plant it in a pot or dedicated plot. There are also various forms of lemon balm supplements, including an encapsulated, powdered extract and a liquid tincture.

I consider lemon balm for pediatric patients with mild anxiety symptoms. It's gentle enough for children but potent enough for most adults to note its calming effects. Validating its long historical use as a nervine, clinical research has confirmed its stress-relieving effects.[10]

If anxiety is more pronounced or longstanding, kava (*Piper methysticum*) is a powerful herbal sedative and anxiolytic. I consider kava for patients who have anxiety that seems random and heightens without an obvious trigger. This characteristic "free-floating anxiety" can be a sign of developmental trauma that is deeply lodged in procedural memory and has not yet found expression in declarative memory.

Kava has been studied in a placebo-controlled, double-blind crossover trial and was found to have significant anxiolytic and antidepressant activity, supporting its traditional use for these conditions.[11]

One final noteworthy herb that is not without its fair share of controversy is cannabis. While many will not respond well to the psychoactive cannabinoid tetrahydrocannabinol (THC), clinical research has documented several medicinal properties of THC and other cannabinoids, such as cannabidiol (CBD).

Pertinent to this discussion is the ability of cannabis to inhibit excitatory neurotransmitters in the amygdala in human studies and increase activity of the prefrontal cortex in animal studies.[12] Thus, cannabis is on the short list as a viable intervention for PTSD, although the benefits are still in question.

Cannabis is being studied in a phase 2 randomized placebo-controlled, double-blind, parallel study to assess safety and efficacy in military veterans diagnosed with PTSD. The results of the trial await publication upon completion.

Cannabis isn't without its obvious downsides. It can be psychologically addictive, disrupt normal REM (dream) sleep with chronic use, and (ironically) induce anxiety and paranoia in some individuals. The hybridization of cannabis plants for recreational use is partly responsible for these negative effects, as such plants contain very high levels of THC. The counterbalancing cannabinoid that hedges for this effect is CBD. Medical marijuana dispensaries offer cannabis that is hybridized to have varying amounts of these two compounds, in some cases offering cannabis strains that contain equal amounts of THC and CBD.

For those seeking guidance on cannabis as medicine, connect with a physician open to and educated on the pros and cons of different preparations of cannabis. In states with medical marijuana dispensaries, full-spectrum cannabis extracts are available for oral use and have seen widespread use by cancer patients dealing with the side effects of conventional oncology treatment.

None of these herbs directly address trauma, but their strength lies in helping build resilience in preparation for the inner work detailed up to this point. To calm the nervous system in the face of trauma is no small feat, so access to these natural substances is a boon to smooth out the bumps on the road to healing trauma.

My comfort zone as a holistic medical provider is to leverage herbs, juxtaposing the fact that I am not a physician with prescribing rights. That said, I would be remiss in failing to acknowledge that psychiatric medications, such as selective serotonin reuptake inhibitors (SSRIs), have a role to play in softening the effects of trauma. However helpful, SSRIs are not panaceas.

"After conducting numerous studies of medications for PTSD, I have come to realize that psychiatric medications have a serious down side, as they may deflect attention from dealing with the underlying issues," said van der Kolk, from the perspective of a psychiatrist and researcher. "The brain-disease model takes control over people's fate out of their own hands and puts doctors and insurance companies in charge of fixing their problems."[13]

This is important to keep in mind regardless of whether the remedy is a plant or a drug. In a harm-reduction model of mental health care, providers would educate patients about all available treatment options and create a plan for slowly reducing the use of herbal and pharmaceutical interventions as the benefits of other therapies accrue. Psychiatric medications can be addictive, but it is also possible to have a psychological dependance on substances such as cannabis and ketamine, so their use must come under the watchful eye of skilled psychiatrists.

13

JOURNEYING THROUGH TRAUMA

"If we do not make time for grief, it will not simply disappear. Grief is stubborn. It will make itself heard or we will die trying to silence it. If we don't face it directly it comes out sideways, in ways that aren't always recognizable as grief: explosive anger, uncontrollable anxiety, compulsive shallowness, brooding bitterness, unchecked addiction. Grief is a ghost that can't be put to rest until its purpose has been fulfilled."

—Tish Harrison Warren, from *Prayer in the Night*

Yet another way to define trauma is as an unexperienced experience. Consider a trauma that causes dissociation, the pain so great that we detach from an aspect of ourselves as a defense mechanism. Whatever the extent and breadth of that separation, the outcome is that trauma has not been assimilated in any meaningful way.

Dissociation is viewed by wisdom traditions among ancestral peoples as a loss of personal power. Recovering from trauma entails retrieval of that portion of one's power left behind at the site of trauma to complete the healing process. Spiritual healing is the purview of ritual and prayer and takes many forms, depending on the culture and its religious beliefs. Let's first explore the ancestral practice of shamanism.

Shamanism is the oldest healing and spiritual practice in the world. Passed on by generations of indigenous healers, the rituals and practices of shamanic medicine are as diverse as the cultures from which they've arisen.

While unbroken ancestral lineages of shamanic practice still exist, modern practitioners of shamanism pull from different traditions. The common elements of shamanic practice include a fluency in some form of divination to diagnose a spiritual imbalance and a means to realize healing.

The diagnosis aspect entails entering an altered state of consciousness. Though methods vary depending on the tradition, ranging from a psychedelic plant medicine to ritual dancing, modern shamans almost exclusively rely on the entraining rhythm of a drum or rattle. Once in that liminal space, the shaman consults with his or her spirit guides to help diagnose when, why, and how an individual or tribe has lost its power.

There are many ways we lose our personal power, but the

concept of a fracturing of the soul is most pertinent to a discussion on trauma and cancer. Physical or emotional trauma may result in a spiritual form of illness known as soul loss.

It is the job of the shaman to divine the nature of the soul loss and then act as an intermediary to bring the lost portion of the soul back to the individual to restore wholeness. Traditionally, this might have involved rituals with dance, song, music, plant medicine, or a combination thereof. Modern shamanic counselors are taught to retrieve the lost portion of the soul while journeying and to "seal" the work in a healing ceremony. Homework is often given to help the client integrate the part and allow it to be fully expressed.

For those who have availed themselves of shamanic healing from an experienced practitioner, the results can be life changing, though it can be a culturally challenging proposition for the person who has never stepped outside of modern Western culture. For such an individual, the ritual fanfare of shamanism may get relegated to an archaic practice of psychodrama.

This wasn't the case for me. Traditional Chinese medicine acknowledges spiritual illness, so I had a clear frame of reference for the potential of shamanic intervention. After my experience consulting with a shaman, I also can't argue with results.

This is the promise of shamanism, and I think a great use case for shamanic practice is the reclaiming of one's personal power following the trauma of a cancer diagnosis.

A Healing Shamanic Journey

Core shamanism is an amalgam of techniques derived from many indigenous cultures, taught as a process of personal development. I took a class on shamanism during graduate school. Although I can't recall the specifics, the thrust of the seminar was to learn how to enter an altered state of consciousness with the aid of rhythmic drumming. This is a common practice in revival shamanism as taught by anthropologist Michael Harner who popularized the technique in the West. Listening to an audio track of rhythmic drumming is how I practiced shamanic journeying for years. Thus, the concept was not foreign to me when I booked an appointment with author and shaman Jane Burns.

On a beautiful fall morning, I logged into an online video conference with Jane to experience firsthand what a modern, Western-educated shaman can teach me about trauma. What transpired during that two-hour session was one of the most profound awakening experiences of all the therapies I describe in this book.

During the first few minutes, Jane explained her process of identifying one's social conditioning that, as she puts it, results in a "suppression of the human soul and its own unique yearnings." The goal is to reclaim authenticity, with shamanic journeying comprising the divination aspect of the session and shamanic healing that integrates what is learned from the journey.

With drum in hand, Jane closed her eyes and began to beat out a steady rhythm at a frequency that entrains the brain into the lower range of theta waves. For the next ninety minutes, with her eyes closed the entire time, Jane would drum for periods of time in consultation with her spiritual helpers to divine information on impediments to the full expression of my being.

Occasionally Jane would stop drumming, convey her

findings, and check on their relevance to my stated intention for the session. It was here that Jane painted a picture of early childhood emotional repression that stunted my creative voice and expression. She commented that much of that had been remedied (by necessity) from my cancer diagnosis and healing, but still offered homework to further expand my emotional awareness and creativity.

This was the cornerstone of her assessment. She then scanned my body to detect where emotional repression was exerting its influence. The energy center surrounding my throat was identified, as well as unprocessed emotions—both my own and from empathic contact with others—stuck in my lymph. For someone diagnosed with lymphoma to be told that emotions appeared as unprocessed "sludge" in my lymph system was eye opening.

This body scan dovetailed into extraction work to remove the accumulation of stuck emotions. An "extraction" involves the removal of intrusive energy that doesn't belong to the individual and that can cause both physical and emotional illness.

The next phase was to identify a loss of soul that occurred between the ages of 7 and 9. According to Jane, my soul loss involved seeing injustice and cruelty but being powerless to stop it. Within my physical body, this manifested as an imbalance in my left shoulder that protected my heart from being wounded.

The soul loss was addressed by the process of soul retrieval; Jane reintegrated this lost part into my being at the end of the session. My homework was (and is) to acknowledge that I have witnessed negativity within conformity and to reclaim my own authentic way of being separate from familial and cultural norms.

Just before that, Jane spoke with and provided a message from a power animal. I thought this was going to be the most mundane aspect of the session as I had spent years interfacing with plant and animal spirit guides in hundreds of shamanic sessions.

What happened next still fills me with awe as I recall the memory.

Jane stopped drumming to inform me that the spirit of Owl came through to give me the message that in this life, I will have to walk through a certain amount of darkness, and I will need to see—and speak—through it. The Owl's gift to me was the ability to see through the darkness.

It was at this point that I completely broke down in tears.

What Jane did not and could not know was where exactly my mind went the moment she said "owl." A little over a year prior, I was hospitalized because of a severe small bowel obstruction. Before being admitted, I spent a long night in excruciating pain, periodically vomiting until there was nothing left in me. On that night, lying on the bathroom floor in an exhausted stupor, I focused on one thing that kept me sane. With the window slightly cracked, I heard an owl hooting in the woods behind our home. For some time, that owl hooted, and I used its call to distract me from the suffering I was enduring.

When Jane spoke of seeing through the darkness, I knew exactly what that meant, and I shared this story with her at the close of our session. That was the single most reclaiming message Jane could have provided to help me heal from the trauma of that experience. Internalizing the message, I have changed the narrative surrounding that painful episode from unresolved trauma to one where higher spiritual forces were present, bearing witness with compassion and grace.

Prayer

Prayer is a palette of many colors. To call upon a higher power for guidance, intervention, and forgiveness, or to express gratitude or veneration is most closely associated with monotheistic faiths.

Prayer has a modern psychological twist with the practices of positive affirmation, gratitude journaling, and self-hypnosis. In essence, these practices offer a secular means to center and calm the mind in order to derive meaningful information. Collectively, we can call these practices different types of contemplative prayer.

Whether someone achieves an inward connection via communion with a deity or deeper aspects of human consciousness (or both) is beside the point. What is relevant to a cancer patient healing from trauma is the validation of the experience and the wisdom gleaned.

As part of my cancer-healing journey, I opted for several sessions of an immunotherapy drug via intravenous infusion. Before my first session, I was informed of the acute side effects that may occur due to the dramatic immune response known as tumor lysis syndrome. Sure enough, as the monoclonal antibodies began potently targeting mutated lymph cells, my teeth started chattering as whole-body chills rapidly set in. A drop of dosage in the immunotherapy drug and a syringe of steroids later, the symptoms stabilized, and I was able to complete the several-hour infusion.

Even with assurance that there was a decreased likelihood of such a reaction in successive rounds, I decided I would ask permission to pray over the immunotherapy drug before future infusions. The following week, I stated my intentions to the oncology team, and without hesitation, the attending nurse delivered an intravenous bag of the aqueous drug into my hands. She cheerfully offered me as much time as I needed, and I proceeded to get into the "right relationship" with the medication (to borrow a shamanic term).

Closing my eyes in a prayer of contemplation, I centered myself in the moment and set an intention for what I wished to happen next. With gratitude for the wonders of modern medicine, I invited the immunotherapy drug into my energy field and asked that it help heal me with the highest efficacy and without side effects. After a few minutes of offering these thoughts in a peak brain state of gratitude and receptivity, I called the nurse to start the infusion. This was my ritual from the second session through my seventh and last session, after which I was in full remission. I did not experience any side effects from treatment in all those subsequent sessions.

Within a religious context, the invocation of a deity or spiritual intermediary for the benefit of others is called intercessory prayer. Examples include participation in a prayer circle or the laying on of hands over an individual in the name of God.

It takes a village to heal from cancer; the physical needs when recovering from a major illness are many. It also takes a spiritual village, and those who cannot contribute directly to the physical care of a cancer patient can always offer spiritual support. Sometimes you can do both, stirring a pot of soup with healing intentions so that the recipient family can realize spiritual nourishment as much as nutritional.

I was blessed to have many people praying for me during my treatment and recovery. My wife jokes that her parents, a retired Lutheran pastor father and an exemplary pastor's wife mother, have a direct ethernet prayer line to God, while others of shaky faith may be on spotty Wi-Fi. My in-laws are truly remarkable and faithful servants of God, but they would correct this jest by stating that we all have equal and abundant access to grace. In nearly every interaction with my father-in-law since my diagnosis, he hugs me and says, "And remember, Emmanuel," meaning, "God with us."

When I was diagnosed with cancer, my Catholic brother and sister-in-law began a discipline of a saying a daily Hail Mary as an intercessory prayer for my healing. Whether from Catholic or Protestant folded hands, or the prayer rug of my Muslim friends, I am quite sure that all intercessory prayers—for which I am eternally grateful—had their intended effect on my spiritual healing.

How we pray for an individual can matter as much as if we pray. In his book *Healing Words: The Power of Prayer and the Practice of Medicine*, Larry Dossey, MD, offers this insightful passage from reviewing the research on prayer:

> These studies showed clearly that prayer can take many forms. Results occurred not only when people prayed for explicit outcomes, but also when they prayed for nothing specific. Some studies, in fact, showed that a simple "Thy will be done" approach was quantitatively more powerful than when specific results were held in the mind. In many experiments, a simple attitude of prayerfulness—an all-pervading sense of holiness and a feeling of empathy, caring, and compassion for the entity in need—seemed to set the stage for healing.

Dossey goes on to state that he ultimately arrived at a place of not praying for a specific outcome for his patients but to hold a space for the best possible outcome without specifying what "best" meant.

How can we access the power of prayer to heal the wounds of trauma, to find respite from the emotional and psychological torrent of cancer? Prayer can be a catalyst for forgiveness. In some cases, that can be forgiving the perpetrator of a trauma, whether that is a specific person or a generic placeholder such as "terrorists." To be clear, forgiveness is not about condoning or negating the responsibility of the people involved. It is all about accepting that this life-altering event occurred and giving oneself permission to move on. Easier said than done, but in conjunction with the other strategies detailed within these pages, prayer can be one step on a path toward forgiveness.

Prayer is also about letting go. Perhaps the circumstances surrounding a trauma are unresolved. In this instance, prayer can be offered to let go of the false hope that the past will ever change, helping guide thoughts and actions toward a better future. In this way, prayer can help tune the greatest instrument we have for healing change—the insight and inspiration of the Heart-mind. Sometimes that healing change happens spontaneously.

Almost two years after his heart transplant, my father experienced a sudden and radical transformation. Although weaning off his anti-rejection medication to a stable level decreased side effects, he still suffered from fatigue, shakiness, dizziness, and brain fog. Then, in the span of one day—and without any other intervention or recent change in medication—these symptoms markedly disappeared. He described the sensation as a sudden chill running through his body, only it wasn't cold. At the conclusion of the day, his healing was complete, with the aforementioned symptoms never returning.

My dad is at a loss to define what caused this transformation. Was someone in his circle praying fervently for him that morning? Perhaps some deep neurocircuitry started firing again after a period of dormancy? Could it have been an act of grace? Maybe it was all the above? Lacking any precipitating ritual, I have no other language to describe what happened to him other than spontaneous healing.

I hear about these kinds of dramatic transformations from time to time and have had a few of my own. Over the years, several patients have conveyed the experience of a surreal healing dream, often one that contained a deceased relative or friend, and awakening to find a chronic problem completely resolved. I feel no need to rationalize such a profound experience. The fact is, they happen, and maybe we can encourage their occurrence through ritual and prayer.

This begs the question: How does faith play into the spiritual healing of trauma? Sometimes faith is the driving force delivering healing and comfort to a traumatized individual; other times it occurs as an act of grace.

In 1858, an apparition appeared to 14-year-old Bernadette

Soubirous in the grotto of Lourdes in France. The lady clothed in white later identified herself as the Virgin Mary, and after 18 appearances and subsequent investigation by the Catholic church, Lourdes was officially recognized as a sacred site. Decades later, Soubirous was canonized as a saint. Miraculous healings have been attributed to contact with the waters of Lourdes at what is now a Catholic pilgrimage site.

A case study in the power of faith to heal trauma occurs during the annual Warriors to Lourdes initiative. With recent support from the Catholic organization, the Knights of Columbus, the gathering has taken place since 1946 in an international effort to bring together active-duty military and veterans from over 40 countries to heal from the trauma of war. According to the Warriors to Lourdes website:

> During World War II, members of the French military visited the site of St.Bernadette's apparitions, offering prayers for peace. In December of 1944, U.S. military personnel joined British, Belgian, French, and Russian military representatives for a Mass at the Basilica of Our Lady of the Rosary. After the War, French soldiers and their chaplains invited German soldiers and their chaplains to gather to pray together. The purpose of this initiative was to heal physical, emotional, and spiritual wounds and to reconcile the past between these former adversaries by recognizing their common identity as Christians in search of peace.

A segment of the 2014 documentary *Sacred Journeys with Bruce Feiler* follows a group of American soldiers traveling to Lourdes for the annual event. Many went with a heart full of faith, while others harbored doubt, yet all hoped that the communal experience would advance them further down the road of healing the profound trauma experienced during military conflict.

The stories so candidly shared by the participants are not for the faint of heart, but at a site across the river from Lourdes that functions as part hotel and part hospital, the soldiers and veterans ventured forth on a pilgrimage of faith to celebrate Mass and be anointed with the sacred waters of Lourdes.

Whether through the influence and energy of ritual or by the progression of faith into lived experience, something profound occurs in the Heart-mind of those who seek healing in sacred sites such as Lourdes. It may not be physical for those who travel home with their crutches instead of leaving them behind, but the Warriors to Lourdes project is a testament that all can find lasting healing from trauma. This occurs through the peace of sacred space, the support of community, and the sharing of stories that convey the power of vulnerability.

By definition, faith implies doubt. In the absence of doubt, we categorize our experience as knowledge. To experience something that defies explanation and to carry on amidst uncertainty requires faith. A place like Lourdes has miracles attributed to it, verified and documented by the medical team overseeing alleged cures. Still, drinking and bathing in the sacred waters does not guarantee healing. We call such religious observances "mysteries" because we are not yet privy to the reason behind such miracles.

Whether you choose to believe or are skeptical of the influence of divine intervention, the gift of faith is an exercise in surrender. Bad things happen to good people, and trauma begets trauma. But even as pain is a hallmark of the human experience, how we interface with that pain and experience suffering is subjective. Faith, prayer, and ritual all can be a bridge to peace for those who choose to walk across it.

To round out this chapter on spiritual healing, it is worth looking back at all the strategies covered. They may seem like a disparate buffet of options, but there are commonalities. Cognitive strategies, such as meditation, psychotherapy, and neurofeedback, access the executive function of the brain and build stress resilience. These therapies are well documented for their effectiveness in decreasing arousal of the amygdala and balancing the autonomic nervous system.

Somatic therapies such as dance, qigong, and Somatic Experiencing give expression to unconscious, visceral sensations through intuitive awareness. They provide a safe means to bring buried emotional pain to the surface without the need for conscious reflection. Sometimes psychotherapy is overwhelming, carrying the risk of additional trauma through flashbacks. Here, somatic therapies are well suited.

Other therapies, such as EMDR and meridian tapping, help soften the effects of trauma by leveraging declarative memory to help rationalize a healing narrative around traumatic events. These therapies bridge cognitive and somatic therapies by combining psychotherapy with some form of physical, often bilateral, stimulation of the body.

What is fundamental to all these therapies is this notion of bridging the disconnect between bodily sensation and distressing thoughts. I will again defer to the wisdom of Dr. Robert Scaer in his book, *The Body Bears the Burden*, where he describes a woman with a bilateral injury to the amygdala who lacked the capacity to experience fear:

> One conclusion that we can make from this regarding trauma therapy is that we need to down-regulate or shut down the amygdala while the patient images, or otherwise accesses the somatic sensations linked to the traumatic event. Without the amygdala "online" the somatic feelings of arousal will not occur, and implicit procedural memories of the trauma—body sensations and emotionally linked declarative memories—will no longer have a meaning of threat in the present moment of their perception.

To revisit a thread that runs through this book, the modalities of holistic and traditional medicine do not assume a separation of body and mind. Although a disconnect between the two would imply they are distinct entities, it is a false dichotomy born out of Western-reductionist thinking.

It is my opinion that this divide between body and mind stems from one thing: the loss of our connection to the spiritual dimension of life. It is our spiritual essence, what TCM calls the shen and what I've been calling the Heart-mind, that bridges this illusory separation.

Disconnecting the concepts of body, mind, and spirit for ease of discussion does a great disservice to adopting a holistic healing paradigm. Rather, it is more accurate to look at these entities as facets of a human being that can become fractured by trauma. If unresolved, that fracture can run deep. We label those fractures with diagnoses such as PTSD, anxiety, or even heart disease and cancer, but they are all maladaptive expressions of a being struggling to find wholeness.

It is only from a place of deep societal trauma that we lead with the notion that body, mind, and spirit are separate, that the onus of healing rests solely with the individual and not with our relationship with others, and that we are out of balance with nature instead of seeing ourselves as the miraculous amalgam of soil and stardust that we are.

CONCLUSION

"We must never forget that we may also find meaning in life even when confronted with a hopeless situation, when facing fate that cannot be changed. For what then matters is to bear witness to the uniquely human potential at its best, which is to transform a personal tragedy into triumph, to turn one's predicament into a human achievement. When we are no longer able to change the situation—just think of an incurable disease such as inoperable cancer—we are challenged to change ourselves."

—Viktor E. Frankl, from *Man's Search for Meaning*

Dr. Arianne Missimer wanted more than to survive cancer, she wanted to thrive—and thrive she has. Now a successful medical provider and happily married to the love of her life, Arianne is a shining light of resilience, but it took some hard work to get there.

A grueling regimen of chemotherapy rendered Arianne unable

to get off the couch on some days. But not one to be defeated, she did the only reasonable thing for a trained physical therapist: On the days she could pick herself up off the couch, she also picked up her kettlebell. In her memoir, I read a sentiment that perfectly summarizes how we each need to reclaim our power in the face of trauma, in the presence of cancer: "As long as I was holding that kettlebell, cancer would have no control over me."

Those initial workouts were difficult for Arianne, but they were a symbol as much as an exercise in her empowerment. She thrived on movement, so movement became an integral part of healing holistically.

Later in her recovery, Arianne again did the only reasonable thing for a physical therapist to do: She trained for and appeared on the television series *American Ninja Warrior*. Yet the power of her story is not what was happening on the outside but the healing that was occurring on the inside.

In her own, beautiful words:

In the heart of all that, something else remarkable was happening. Not only was my body starting to get stronger and fight back against the horrific disease that had taken so many lives and had tried to take mine…I also felt my old self coming back, I was winning in every possible way: physically, emotionally, and spiritually. It was so incredible just how great I was feeling.

My first memories of this life were in a hospital. Born with two fingers of my left hand webbed together, I had three operations between the ages of 3 and 4 to separate them. I can't recall the emotional content of those fragmented images with any detail, save for the general feeling of anxiety and trepidation.

My family surely has a different perception of those events. My older brother recalls his experience of my stitches being removed. Hearing me wail in pain and fear, it was as traumatic for him sitting in the waiting room as it presumably was for me experiencing it. Thankfully, I don't remember that incident.

The point is that with the best of intentions from all involved, and even with a successful outcome (I'm typing these words with ten fingers), trauma can often be an unintended consequence. Compassionate care can lessen the painful memories associated with traumatic events, but it does not eliminate their influence. Receiving a cancer diagnosis is like that.

Moreover, many endure trauma that occurs without immediate access to support. Childhood abuse can go on for years with some victims not finding solace until adulthood. I wish I could wave a magic wand and take all this pain away from those who have suffered. The best I can do is to foster a dialogue, acknowledging the missing link in health care.

It may never be possible to design a research study demonstrating that early sexual abuse leads to adult-onset diabetes, that rejection can cause irritable bowel syndrome, or that grief can underlie breast cancer formation—but I can prove without a single research dollar that these traumatic events have a tremendous impact on health and well-being.

Stress and trauma shape our perception of the world and the ability to feel safe within it. In the absence of security, many turn to addictions. It could be smoking cigarettes that cause lung cancer or sugary desserts that lead to obesity and diabetes—gateways to hormone-driven malignancies such as ovarian, breast, and pro-state cancer.

These are straightforward examples, but I am just as interested in the subtle stresses and traumas that frame our day-to-day experience. In a modern world obsessed with technology and better living through chemistry, we need a new ethic that honors thoughts and emotions as much as objects.

There are many explanations for and descriptions of the origin of cancer, but perhaps the most revealing, as discussed in this book's introduction, is that of a wound that isn't healing. Implicit in that definition is the understanding that malignancy has a root cause that develops into a chronic imbalance.

In one instance, a carcinogenic exposure may persist over years, damaging DNA faster than the body can repair it. This is the case with radiation exposure or smoking. Another possibility is a single event that creates the seed of cancer that grows under the influence of other proximate causes. This may very well be the case with trauma.

Does this mean trauma causes cancer? This book is not about validating that statement. Rather, it's about taking a holistic perspective on health and disease. Trauma is, unequivocally, a major underlying cause of ill health. Whether trauma is a textbook carcinogen is beside the point.

Consider stress, the subject of one of my previous books. After publication, many readers inquired whether I thought stress is a cause of cancer, perhaps because I never made that explicit claim. My answer is that chronic stress is a potent proximate cause of cancer, suggesting that it strongly promotes cancer growth that has been initiated by some other means.

This does not imply that the damaging influence of stress should be ignored simply because it is not the root cause of cancer. Removing the initiating carcinogen is always best, but if it cannot be addressed, we have no choice but to mitigate the proximate causes that are feeding cancer growth. This is the terrain theory of addressing the cancer microenvironment, bolstering the resilience of the body-mind and instilling the resolve to maintain a healthy, anticancer lifestyle for years to come.

Returning to the pond analogy from Chapter 1, stress is akin to throwing small pebbles in the pond of life. The ripples of chronic stress can wear down one's resilience and open the door to chronic illness. Trauma is different; it is a boulder that displaces water from the pond. This is how trauma, as a single incident, can have repercussions throughout one's life. Mitigating chronic stress requires lifestyle adjustments; healing trauma requires restoring the primacy of the Heart-mind. In the absence of our personal power, the seed of cancer can take root.

If trauma is in fact a root cause of cancer, then a profound opportunity for empowerment is available to all those brave enough to do the work. Healing past trauma means to address a root cause of illness, one that underlies addictions, destructive behaviors, and feeling unsafe or unwanted on planet earth. If cancer is a wound that isn't healing, then trauma would be chief among the wounding events.

A correlation between trauma and cancer incidence may be just that, a correlation. The weight of the evidence presented here is compelling but not absolute. It may be some time before science can answer this question with any degree of certainty. Yet the wise cancer patient, caregiver, or oncologist can read the writing on the wall (or in this book) and take away an actionable means of deep, life-changing healing.

Just like stress, even if trauma were a proximate cause to carcinogenic exposure, it should be addressed with compassion and determination. The future of oncology care should be—hopefully will be—equally vested in health as in disease. There will always be a place for anticancer strategies such as drugs or herbs, but adherence to an anticancer lifestyle is the missing piece of the puzzle. With advances in oncology, and a personal journey of returning to wholeness, it may very well be possible to live with cancer but not die from it. With that mindset, cancer will not be a tragedy from which we succumb, but a friend and wise teacher who guides us back on the path of meaning and empowerment.

Memento mori is Latin for "Remember death." It is a phrase used as a reminder that death is near, so appreciate your life. I recently learned of its use at a Catholic monastery. Every night, one chosen monk is responsible for walking the halls of the other monks' living quarters to bang on each door and shout "*Memento mori!*" That's a wake-up call on many levels.

If you have been diagnosed with cancer, you no doubt get daily reminders of your mortality, and that can be a good thing if you let it change you. Yet some are quick to forget the trials of the experience. The word "remission" or the phrases "pathological complete response" or "no evidence of disease" lull us back into complacency. We forget about death at the risk of losing touch with that which brings life. Or we struggle with the opposite, ruminating on the damage done and the suffering that might still occur.

I ceased pretending to be strong a long time ago. My body is broken—it is being held together by faith and radical acceptance. I've also come to realize that positive and negative emotions are not mutually exclusive. Fear of cancer relapse and grief for the loss perpetrated by cancer haven't gone away; I've just learned to leave room for other emotions. The fear, worry, and grief are as much a part of me as the joyous experiences of life, and I weave all those emotions together into a rope that pulls me forward toward truth and empowerment.

I recommend every cancer patient consider a daily practice of contemplating a different mantra: "*Memento vitae!*" or "Remember life!" By that I don't mean recall a time in your life before cancer or before trauma. For some people, that might not be possible.

Instead, remember the possibilities of life. Remember that forgiveness is less about the other person and more about what you choose to feel in your Heart-mind. Remember that a sublime ocean of peace is available to you—even with your last breath— if you just let go. Remember that there is a place deep within that no malignancy can ever metastasize to, a place beyond the ravages of any disease. That is the life and light from which you came and to which you return.

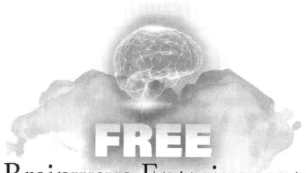

FREE
Brainwave Entrainment
Meditation
for newsletter subscribers!

www.CancerMindset.com

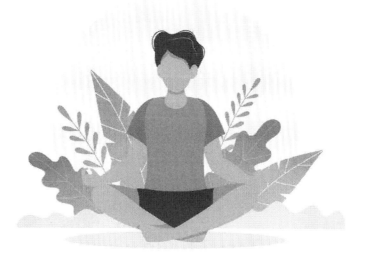

ACKNOWLEDGMENTS

If the Lorax speaks for the trees, I wish to be known as the spokesperson for unsung heroes. Praise is liberally given to those in the spotlight, but the fabric of a healthy society is held together by the quiet peacemakers working behind the scenes. Women are often the thankless nurturers of that cohesion, and in the story of my life, three such women have played a central role and are the lifelong recipients of my gratitude. I will extend my appreciation to them in the order we became acquainted:

To my mother, Rita LaGreca—you have endured much in life but had the strength and courage to transcend your history and provide a safe and stable home for your children. You broke cycles of abuse that could easily have been passed on, but your Heart-mind saw a better life for your children, and we have realized it thanks to your compassion and forbearance. That is a debt that can only be paid forward, as it is being done now in the vibrant lives of your grandchildren.

Even though we are far apart, our innate connection, forged with love, transcends time and space. Because you understand that, I rest in the peaceful realization that we are never apart.

To my mentor, Natalie "Karina" Arndt—I can't thank you enough for taking me under your wing. You gave my clinical career a strong foundation, and it is not an exaggeration to state that there is a little piece of your shen in all the patients I treat.

There is a Greek Stoic tale that if everyone put their worries in a communal pool and extracted an equal portion, most people would be happier enduring what they originally had. You are one of those who would take the trade and be better for it. That you have lived an inspiring life of service despite the burden you carry is a testament to your resilience. And please forgive me for not putting a section on Nonviolent Communication in this book.

To my wife, Joy Hernes—you get the award for unsung hero in the caregiver role. Cancer took as much from you emotionally as it did from me physically. The years following have been filled with uncertainty, but you have spared our daughter from the worst of the fallout. I'm sorry for all that you have had to go through and thank you for being my safe person. In everything I write about cancer, there is an element of your story woven within. To all who acknowledge my work with gratitude, please also honor Joy for being chief among those who have enabled me to share the message of empowerment. *Omnia vincit amor et nos cedamus amori.*

Much of the manuscript for this book was written while listening to the album *Light for the World* by the Poor Claire Sisters of Arundel. Thank you for your light, Sisters.

ABOUT THE AUTHOR

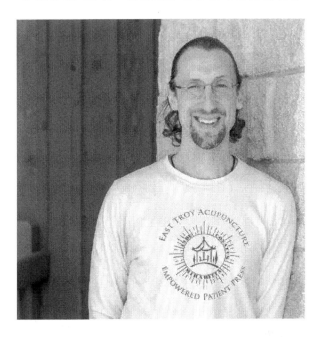

Brandon LaGreca, LAc, MAcOM, grew up on the East Coast of the U.S. and attended Montclair State University, where he received a bachelor's degree in science with a minor in religion, summa cum laude. He then moved to the West Coast to fulfill a dream he had from the age of 12 of studying traditional Chinese medicine. He was accepted to the prestigious Oregon College of Oriental Medicine, where he earned a master's degree in acupuncture and Oriental medicine. His postgraduate work included studying and working at Nanjing University of Chinese Medicine in China.

After 10 years of private practice, Brandon experienced first-hand the journey of the wounded healer when a series of small bowel obstructions led to hospitalization and diagnosis of stage 4 non-Hodgkin's lymphoma. He achieved remission eight months later following an integrative oncology protocol that included immunotherapy without surgery, radiation, or chemotherapy. He now lectures and writes on the epigenetics of cancer and has dedicated his career to empowering patients through and beyond chronic illnesses such as cancer. His latest interests include studying indigenous forms of healing and eco-spirituality.

He is also the author of *Cancer and EMF Radiation: How to Protect Yourself From the Silent Carcinogen of Electropollution* and *Cancer, Stress & Mindset: Focusing the Mind to Empower Healing and Resilience*. He shares his thoughts at

EmpoweredPatientBlog.com

REFERENCES

Chapter 1

1. Mukherjee, Siddhartha. *The Emperor of All Maladies: A Biography of Cancer*. Simon & Schuster, 2011.
2. Damasio, Antonio R., Thomas J. Grabowski, Antoine Bechara, Hanna Damasio, Laura L.B. Ponto, Josef Parvizi, and Richard D. Hichwa. "Subcortical and Cortical Brain Activity during the Feeling of Self-Generated Emotions." *Nature Neuro-science* 3, no. 10 (October 1, 2000): 1049–56. https://doi.org/10.1038/79871.
3. Seal, Karen H., Daniel Bertenthal, Christian R. Miner, Saunak Sen, and Charles Marmar. "Bringing the War Back Home: Mental Health Disorders Among 103 788 US Veterans Returning From Iraq and Afghanistan Seen at Department of Veterans Affairs Facilities." *Archives of Internal Medicine* 167, no. 5 (March 12, 2007): 476–82. https://doi.org/10.1001/archinte.167.5.476.
4. Hoge, Charles W., Jennifer L. Auchterlonie, and Charles S. Milliken. "Mental Health Problems, Use of Mental Health Services, and Attrition From Military Service After Returning From Deployment to Iraq or Afghanistan." *JAMA* 295, no. 9 (March 1, 2006): 1023–32. https://doi.org/10.1001/jama.295.9.1023.
5. Rosenberg, Stanley. *Accessing the Healing Power of the Vagus Nerve: Self-Help Exercises for Anxiety, Depression, Trauma, and Autism*. North Atlantic Books, 2017.

6. Roberts, Andrea L., Tianyi Huang, Karestan C. Koenen, Yongjoo Kim, Laura D. Kubzansky, and Shelley S. Tworoger. "Posttraumatic Stress Disorder Is Associated with Increased Risk of Ovarian Cancer: A Prospective and Retrospective Longitudinal Cohort Study." *Cancer Research* 79, no. 19 (October 1, 2019): 5113–20. https://doi.org/10.1158/0008-5472.CAN-19-1222.

Chapter 2

1. Kolk, Bessel A van der, Mark S Greenberg, Scott P Orr, and RK Pitman. "Endogenous Opioids, Stress Induced Analgesia, and Posttraumatic Stress Disorder." *Psychopharmacology Bulletin* 25, no. 3 (1989): 417–21.
2. Van der Kolk, Bessel. "The Body Keeps the Score: Brain, Mind, and Body in the Healing of Trauma." *New York*, 2014.
3. Kolk, Bessel A. van der, and Rita Fisler. "Dissociation and the Fragmentary Nature of Traumatic Memories: Overview and Exploratory Study." *Journal of Traumatic Stress* 8, no. 4 (October 1, 1995): 505–25. https://doi.org/10.1007/BF02102887.
4. ——— "The Body Keeps the Score: Brain, Mind, and Body in the Healing of Trauma." *New York*, 2014.
5. ——— "The Body Keeps the Score: Brain, Mind, and Body in the Healing of Trauma." *New York*, 2014.
6. U.S. Department of Health and Human Services, Administration for Children and Families, Administration on Children, Youth and Families, Children's Bureau. *Child Maltreatment 2010.*

Washington, DC: U.S. Government Printing Office, 2011. Accessed September 16, 2023. https://www.acf.hhs.gov/cb/report/child-maltreatment-2020.

7. Christopher, Michael. "A Broader View of Trauma: A Biopsychosocial-Evolutionary View of the Role of the Traumatic Stress Response in the Emergence of Pathology and/or Growth." *Clinical Psychology Review* 24, no. 1 (March 1, 2004): 75–98. https://doi.org/10.1016/j.cpr.2003.12.003.

8. Teicher, Martin H., Susan L. Andersen, Ann Polcari, Carl M. Anderson, and Carryl P. Navalta. "Developmental Neurobiology of Childhood Stress and Trauma." *Psychiatric Clinics of North America* 25, no. 2 (June 1, 2002): 397–426. https://doi.org/10.1016/S0193-953X(01)00003-X.

9. "Evoked Potential Evidence for Right Brain Activity during the Recall of Traumatic Memories." *The Journal of Neuropsychiatry and Clinical Neurosciences* 7, no. 2 (May 1, 1995): 169–75. https://doi.org/10.1176/jnp.7.2.169.

10. Teicher, Martin H., Susan L. Andersen, Ann Polcari, Carl M. Anderson, and Carryl P. Navalta. "Developmental Neurobiology of Childhood Stress and Trauma." *Psychiatric Clinics of North America* 25, no. 2 (June 1, 2002): 397–426. https://doi.org/10.1016/S0193-953X(01)00003-X.

11. American Cancer Society. "Family Cancer Syndromes." Accessed May 5, 2023. https://www.cancer.org/cancer/risk-prevention/genetics/family-cancer-syndromes.html.

12. Morgan, Hugh D., Heidi G.E. Sutherland, David I.K. Martin, and Emma Whitelaw. "Epigenetic Inheritance at the Agouti Locus in the Mouse." *Nature Genetics* 23, no. 3 (November 1,

1999): 314–18. https://doi.org/10.1038/15490.

13. Yehuda, Rachel, Nikolaos P. Daskalakis, Linda M. Bierer, Heather N. Bader, Torsten Klengel, Florian Holsboer, and Elisabeth B. Binder. "Holocaust Exposure Induced Intergenerational Effects on FKBP5 Methylation." *Corticotropin-Releasing Factor, FKBP5, and Posttraumatic Stress Disorder* 80, no. 5 (September 1, 2016): 372–80. https://doi.org/10.-1016/j.biopsych.2015.08.005.

14. Bierer, Linda M., Heather N. Bader, Nikolaos P. Daskalakis, Amy Lehrner, Nadine Provençal, Tobias Wiechmann, Torsten Klengel, Iouri Makotkine, Elisabeth B. Binder, and Rachel Yehuda. "Intergenerational Effects of Maternal Holocaust Exposure on FKBP5 Methylation." *American Journal of Psychiatry* 177, no. 8 (August 1, 2020): 744–53. https://doi.org/10.1176/appi.ajp.2019.19060618.

15. Daskalakis, Nikolaos P., Changxin Xu, Heather N. Bader, Chris Chatzinakos, Peter Weber, Iouri Makotkine, Amy Lehrner, Linda M. Bierer, Elisabeth B. Binder, and Rachel Yehuda. "Intergenerational Trauma Is Associated with Expression Alterations in Glucocorticoid- and Immune-Related Genes." *Neuropsychopharmacology* 46, no. 4 (March 1, 2021): 763–73. https://doi.org/10.1038/s41386-020-00900-8.

16. LaGreca, Brandon. *Cancer, Stress & Mindset: Focusing the Mind to Empower Healing and Resilience.* Empowered Patient Press, 2021.

17. Yehuda, Rachel, Stephanie Mulherin Engel, Sarah R. Brand, Jonathan Seckl, Sue M. Marcus, and Gertrud S. Berkowitz. "Transgenerational Effects of Posttraumatic Stress Disorder in

Babies of Mothers Exposed to the World Trade Center Attacks during Pregnancy." *The Journal of Clinical Endo-crinology & Metabolism* 90, no. 7 (July 1, 2005): 4115–18. https://doi.org/10.1210/jc.2005-0550.

18. Lupien, Sonia J., Bruce S. McEwen, Megan R. Gunnar, and Christine Heim. "Effects of Stress throughout the Lifespan on the Brain, Behaviour and Cognition." *Nature Reviews Neuroscience* 10, no. 6 (June 1, 2009): 434–45. https://doi.org/10.1038/nrn2639.

19. Dickson, David A., Jessica K. Paulus, Virginia Mensah, Janis Lem, Lorena Saavedra-Rodriguez, Adrienne Gentry, Kelly Pagidas, and Larry A. Feig. "Reduced Levels of MiRNAs 449 and 34 in Sperm of Mice and Men Exposed to Early Life Stress." *Translational Psychiatry* 8, no. 1 (May 23, 2018): 101. https://doi.org/10.1038/s41398-018-0146-2.

20. Yehuda, Rachel, Sarah L. Halligan, and Robert Grossman. "Childhood Trauma and Risk for PTSD: Relationship to Intergenerational Effects of Trauma, Parental PTSD, and Cortisol Excretion." *Development and Psychopathology* 13, no. 3 (2001): 733–53. https://doi.org/10.1017/S0954579401003170.

21. Franklin, Tamara B., Holger Russig, Isabelle C. Weiss, Johannes Gräff, Natacha Linder, Aubin Michalon, Sandor Vizi, and Isabelle M. Mansuy. "Epigenetic Transmission of the Impact of Early Stress Across Generations." *Stress, Neuroplasticity, and Posttraumatic Stress Disorder* 68, no. 5 (September 1, 2010): 408–15. https://doi.org/10.1016/j.biopsych.2010.05.036.

22. Franklin, Tamara B., Holger Russig, Isabelle C. Weiss, Johannes Gräff, Natacha Linder, Aubin Michalon, Sandor Vizi, and Isabelle M. Mansuy. "Epigenetic Transmission of the Impact of Early Stress Across Generations." *Stress, Neuroplasticity, and Posttraumatic Stress Disorder* 68, no. 5 (September 1, 2010): 408–15. https://doi.org/10.1016/j.biopsych.2010.05.036.

23. Dias, Brian G, and Kerry J Ressler. "Parental Olfactory Experience Influences Behavior and Neural Structure in Subsequent Generations." *Nature Neuroscience* 17, no. 1 (January 1, 2014): 89–96. https://doi.org/10.1038/nn.3594.

24. Skinner, Michael K, and Carlos Guerrero-Bosagna. "Environmental Signals and Transgenerational Epigenetics." *Epigenomics* 1, no. 1 (October 1, 2009): 111–17. https://doi.org/10.2217/epi.09.11.

Chapter 3

1. Holt-Lunstad, Julianne, Timothy B. Smith, and J. Bradley Layton. "Social Relationships and Mortality Risk: A Meta-Analytic Review." *PLOS Medicine* 7, no. 7 (July 27, 2010): e1000316. https://doi.org/10.1371/journal.pmed.1000316.

2. Cacioppo, John T., Louise C. Hawkley, L. Elizabeth Crawford, John M. Ernst, Mary H. Burleson, Ray B. Kowalewski, William B. Malarkey, Eve Van Cauter, and Gary G. Berntson. "Loneliness and Health: Potential Mechanisms." *Psychosomatic Medicine* 64, no. 3 (2002). https://journals.lww.com/psychosomaticmedicine/Fulltext/200

2/05000/Loneliness_and_Health__Potential_Mechanisms.5.as
px.

3. Christopher, Michael. "A Broader View of Trauma: A Biopsychosocial-Evolutionary View of the Role of the Traumatic Stress Response in the Emergence of Pathology and/or Growth." *Clinical Psychology Review* 24, no. 1 (March 1, 2004): 75–98. https://doi.org/10.1016/j.cpr.2003.12.003.

4. Siegel, Bernie S. *Love, Medicine and Miracles.* Harper & Row, 1986.

Chapter 4

1. Koenigs, Michael, and Jordan Grafman. "Posttraumatic Stress Disorder: The Role of Medial Prefrontal Cortex and Amygdala." *The Neuroscientist* 15, no. 5 (October 1, 2009): 540–48. https://doi.org/10.1177/1073858409333072

2. LaGreca, Brandon. *Cancer, Stress & Mindset: Focusing the Mind to Empower Healing and Resilience.* Empowered Patient Press, 2021.

3. Van der Kolk, Bessel. "The Body Keeps the Score: Brain, Mind, and Body in the Healing of Trauma." *New York*, 2014.

4. Mason, J. W., Giller, E. L., Kosten, T. R., Ostroff, R. B., & Podd, L. (1986). Urinary free-cortisol levels in posttraumatic stress disorder patients. *Journal of Nervous and Mental Disease, 174*(3), 145–149. https://doi.org/10.1097/00005053-198603000-00003

5. Preston, Graeme, Faisal Kirdar, and Tamas Kozicz. "The Role of Suboptimal Mitochondrial Function in Vulnerability to

Posttraumatic Stress Disorder." *Journal of Inherited Metabolic Disease* 41, no. 4 (July 1, 2018): 585–96. https://doi.org/10.1007/s10545-018-0168-1.

6. Stout, Daniel M., Monte S. Buchsbaum, Andrea D. Spadoni, Victoria B. Risbrough, Irina A. Strigo, Scott C. Matthews, and Alan N. Simmons. "Multimodal Canonical Correlation Reveals Converging Neural Circuitry across Trauma-Related Disorders of Affect and Cognition." *Neurobiology of Stress* 9 (November 1, 2018): 241–50. https://doi.org/10.1016/j.ynstr.2018.09.006.

7. Zantvoord, Jasper B., Paul Zhutovsky, Judith B.M. Ensink, Rosanne Op den Kelder, Guido A. van Wingen, and Ramon J.L. Lindauer. "Trauma-Focused Psychotherapy Response in Youth with Posttraumatic Stress Disorder Is Associated with Changes in Insula Volume." *Journal of Psychiatric Research* 132 (January 1, 2021): 207–14. https://doi.org/10.1016/j.jpsychires.2020.10.037.

8. Brown, David W., Robert F. Anda, Henning Tiemeier, Vincent J. Felitti, Valerie J. Edwards, Janet B. Croft, and Wayne H. Giles. "Adverse Childhood Experiences and the Risk of Premature Mortality." *American Journal of Preventive Medicine* 37, no. 5 (November 1, 2009): 389–96. https://doi.org/10.1016/j.amepre.2009.06.021.

9. Kelly-Irving, Michelle, Benoit Lepage, Dominique Dedieu, Rebecca Lacey, Noriko Cable, Melanie Bartley, David Blane, Pascale Grosclaude, Thierry Lang, and Cyrille Delpierre. "Childhood Adversity as a Risk for Cancer: Findings from the 1958 British Birth Cohort Study." *BMC Public Health* 13, no.

1 (August 19, 2013): 767. https://doi.org/10.1186/1471-2458-13-767.

10. Eysenck, H.J. "Cancer, Personality and Stress: Prediction and Prevention." *Advances in Behaviour Research and Therapy* 16, no. 3 (January 1, 1994): 167–215. https://doi.org/10.1016/0146-6402(94)00001-8.

11. Baltrusch, H. J., W. Stangel, and I. Titze. "Stress, Cancer and Immunity: New Developments in Biopsychosocial and Psychoneuroimmunologic Research." *Acta Neurologica* 13, no. 4 (1991): 315–327. PMID: 1781308.

12. Wirsching, Michael, Helm Stierlin, Florian Hoffmann, Gunthard Weber, and Barbara Wirsching. "Psychological Identification of Breast Cancer Patients before Biopsy." *Journal of Psychosomatic Research* 26, no. 1 (January 1, 1982): 1–10. https://doi.org/10.1016/0022-3999(82)90057-5.

13. Thomas, Sandra P., Maureen Groer, Mitzi Davis, Patricia Droppleman, Johnie Mozingo, and Margaret Pierce. "Anger and Cancer: AN ANALYSIS OF THE LINKAGES." *Cancer Nursing* 23, no. 5 (2000). https://journals.lww.com/cancernursingonline/Fulltext/2000/10000/Anger_and_Cancer__AN_ANALYSIS_OF_THE_LINKAGES.3.aspx.

14. Penedo, Frank J., Jason R. Dahn, Dave Kinsinger, Michael H. Antoni, Ivan Molton, Jeffrey S. Gonzalez, Mary Anne Fletcher, Bernard Roos, Charles S. Carver, and Neil Schneiderman. "Anger Suppression Mediates the Relationship between Optimism and Natural Killer Cell Cytotoxicity in Men Treated for Localized Prostate Cancer." *Journal of Psychosomatic*

Research 60, no. 4 (April 1, 2006): 423–27.
https://doi.org/10.1016/j.jpsychores.2005.08.001.

15. Visintainer Madelon A., Volpicelli Joseph R., and Seligman Martin E. P. "Tumor Rejection in Rats After Inescapable or Escapable Shock." *Science* 216, no. 4544 (April 23, 1982): 437–39. https://doi.org/10.1126/science.7200261.

16. Maier, Steven F, and Martin E Seligman. "Learned Helplessness: Theory and Evidence." *Journal of Experimental Psychology: General* 105, no. 1 (1976): 3. https://doi.org/10.1037/0096-3445.105.1.3.

Chapter 5

1. Dicks, Leon M. T. "Gut Bacteria and Neurotransmitters." *Microorganisms* 10, no. 9 (2022). https://doi.org/10.3390/microorganisms10091838.

2. Mayer, Emeran A. "Gut Feelings: The Emerging Biology of Gut–Brain Communication." *Nature Reviews Neuroscience* 12, no. 8 (August 1, 2011): 453–66. https://doi.org/10.1038/nrn3071.

3. Strandwitz, Philip. "Neurotransmitter Modulation by the Gut Microbiota." *Where the Gut Meets the Brain* 1693 (August 15, 2018): 128–33. https://doi.org/10.1016/j.brainres.2018.03.015.

4. McCraty, Rollin. "The Energetic Heart: Bioelectromagnetic Interactions within and between People." *Boulder Creek, CA: Institute of HeartMath*, 2003.

5. McCraty, Rollin, Mike Atkinson, Dana Tomasino, and Raymond Trevor Bradley. "The Coherent Heart Heart-Brain Interactions, Psychophysiological Coherence, and the Emergence of

System-Wide Order." *Integral Review: A Transdisciplinary & Transcultural Journal for New Thought, Research, & Praxis* 5, no. 2 (2009).

6. M. S. Gazzaniga, The Social Brain: Discovering the Networks of the Mind (New York: Basic Books, 1985), 90.

Chapter 7

1. On Humanity's Emotions and Higher Virtues: A Passage from the Chapter "Qingxing" in the 'Baihu tongde lun' (Discussions on the Power of Virtue in the White Tiger Hall; attributed to Ban Gu). Translated by Heiner Fruehauf.

Part 3—A Path to Healing

1. Hubble, M. A., Duncan, B. L., & Miller, S. D. (Eds.). (1999). *The heart and soul of change: What works in therapy.* American Psychological Association. https://doi.org/10.1037/11132-000.

2. Benish, Steven G., Zac E. Imel, and Bruce E. Wampold. "The Relative Efficacy of Bona Fide Psychotherapies for Treating Posttraumatic Stress Disorder: A Meta-Analysis of Direct Comparisons." *Clinical Psychology Review* 28, no. 5 (June 1, 2008): 746–58. https://doi.org/10.1016/j.cpr.2007.10.005.

Chapter 9

1. Breitbart, William, Hayley Pessin, Barry Rosenfeld, Allison J Applebaum, Wendy G Lichtenthal, Yuelin Li, Rebecca M

Saracino, Allison M Marziliano, Melissa Masterson, and Kristen Tobias. "Individual Meaning-centered Psychotherapy for the Treatment of Psychological and Existential Distress: A Randomized Controlled Trial in Patients with Advanced Cancer." *Cancer* 124, no. 15 (2018): 3231–39. https://doi.org/10.1002/cncr.31539.

2. Thomas, Lori P. Montross, Emily A. Meier, and Scott A. Irwin. "Meaning-Centered Psychotherapy: A Form of Psychotherapy for Patients With Cancer." *Current Psychiatry Reports* 16, no. 10 (September 4, 2014): 488. https://doi.org/10.1007/s11920-014-0488-2.

3. Yehuda, Rachel, Nikolaos Daskalakis, Frank Desarnaud, Iouri Makotkine, Amy Lehrner, Erin Koch, Janine Flory, Joseph Buxbaum, Michael Meaney, and Linda Bierer. "Epigenetic Biomarkers as Predictors and Correlates of Symptom Improvement Following Psychotherapy in Combat Veterans with PTSD." *Frontiers in Psychiatry* 4 (2013). https://doi.org/10.3389/fpsyt.2013.00118.

4. Gapp, Katharina, Johannes Bohacek, Jonas Grossmann, Andrea M Brunner, Francesca Manuella, Paolo Nanni, and Isabelle M Mansuy. "Potential of Environmental Enrichment to Prevent Transgenerational Effects of Paternal Trauma." *Neuropsychopharmacology* 41, no. 11 (October 1, 2016): 2749–58. https://doi.org/10.1038/npp.2016.87.

5. Energy Psychology Journal. "Differential Gene Expression after Emotional Freedom Techniques (EFT) Treatment: A Novel Pilot Protocol for Salivary MRNA Assessment." Accessed February 12, 2020.

https://energypsychologyjournal.org/differential-gene-expression-emotional-freedom-techniques-eft-treatment-novel-pilot-protocol-salivary-mrna-assessment/.

6. Bach, Donna, Gary Groesbeck, Peta Stapleton, Rebecca Sims, Katharina Blickheuser, and Dawson Church. "Clinical EFT (Emotional Freedom Techniques) Improves Multiple Physiological Markers of Health." *Journal of Evidence-Based Integrative Medicine* 24 (January 1, 2019): 2515690X1-8823691. https://doi.org/10.1177/2515690X18823691.

7. Church, Dawson, Oscar Piña, Carla Reategui, and Audrey Brooks. "Single-Session Reduction of the Intensity of Traumatic Memories in Abused Adolescents after EFT: A Randomized Controlled Pilot Study." *Traumatology* 18, no. 3 (2012): 73–79. https://doi.org/10.1177/1534765611426788.

8. Shapiro, Francine, and Deany Laliotis. "EMDR Therapy for Trauma-Related Disorders." In *Evidence Based Treatments for Trauma-Related Psychological Disorders: A Practical Guide for Clinicians*, edited by Ulrich Schnyder and Marylène Cloitre, 205–28. Cham: Springer International Publishing, 2015. https://doi.org/10.1007/978-3-319-07109-1_11.

9. B. A. van der Kolk, et al., "A Randomized Clinical Trial of Eye Movement Desensitization and Reprocessing (EMDR), Fluoxetine, and Pill Placebo in the Treatment of Posttraumatic Stress Disorder: Treatment Effects and Long-Term Maintenance," Journal of Clinical Psychiatry 68, no. 1 (2007): 37–46.

10. World Health Organization. "Guidelines for the Management of Conditions That Are Specifically Related to Stress," 2013. PMID: 24049868.

11. Hodgdon, Hilary B., Frank G. Anderson, Elizabeth Southwell, Wendy Hrubec, and Richard Schwartz. "Internal Family Systems (IFS) Therapy for Posttraumatic Stress Disorder (PTSD) among Survivors of Multiple Childhood Trauma: A Pilot Effectiveness Study." *Journal of Aggression, Maltreatment & Trauma* 31, no. 1 (January 2, 2022): 22–43. https://doi.org/10.1080/10926771.2021.2013375.

Chapter 10

1. Cohen, Hagit, Jonathan Benjamin, Amir B. Geva, Mike A. Matar, Zeev Kaplan, and Moshe Kotler. "Autonomic Dysregulation in Panic Disorder and in Posttraumatic Stress Disorder: Application of Power Spectrum Analysis of Heart Rate Variability at Rest and in Response to Recollection of Trauma or Panic Attacks." *Psychiatry Research* 96, no. 1 (September 25, 2000): 1–13. https://doi.org/10.1016/S0165-1781(00)00195-5.

2. Larsen, Stephen, and Leslie Sherlin. "Neurofeedback: An Emerging Technology for Treating Central Nervous System Dysregulation." *Complementary and Integrative Therapies for Psychiatric Disorders* 36, no. 1 (March 1, 2013): 163–68. https://doi.org/10.1016/j.psc.2013.01.005.

3. Larsen, Stephen. *The Neurofeedback Solution: How to Treat Autism, ADHD, Anxiety, Brain Injury, Stroke, PTSD, and More.* Simon & Schuster, 2012.

4. Fisher, Sebern F. *Neurofeedback in the Treatment of*

Developmental Trauma: Calming the Fear-Driven Brain. WW Norton & Company, 2014.

5. Yamamoto, Shin, Yoshihiro Kitamura, Norihito Yamada, Yoshihiko Nakashima, and Shigetoshi Kuroda. "Medial Prefrontal Cortex and Anterior Cingulate Cortex in the Generation of Alpha Activity Induced by Transcendental Meditation: A Magnetoencephalographic Study." *Acta Medica Okayama* 60, no. 1 (2006): 51–58. http://doi.org/10.18926/AMO/30752.

6. Taren, Adrienne A., J. David Creswell, and Peter J. Gianaros. "Dispositional Mindfulness Co-Varies with Smaller Amygdala and Caudate Volumes in Community Adults." *PLOS ONE* 8, no. 5 (May 22, 2013): e64574. https://doi.org/10.1371/journal.pone.0064574.

7. Davidson, Richard J., Jon Kabat-Zinn, Jessica Schumacher, Melissa Rosenkranz, Daniel Muller, Saki F. Santorelli, Ferris Urbanowski, Anne Harrington, Katherine Bonus, and John F. Sheridan. "Alterations in Brain and Immune Function Produced by Mindfulness Meditation." *Psychosomatic Medicine* 65, no. 4 (2003). http://dx.doi.org/10.1097/01.PSY.0000077505.67574.E3.

8. McCraty, Rollin. "Following the Rhythm of the Heart: HeartMath Institute's Path to HRV Biofeedback." *Applied Psychophysiology and Biofeedback* 47, no. 4 (December 1, 2022): 305–16. https://doi.org/10.1007/s10484-022-09554-2.

9. McCraty, R. "Exploring the Role of the Heart in Human Performance." *Science of the Heart* 2 (2016): 70.

10. Pyne, Jeffrey M, Joseph I Constans, John T Nanney, Mark D

Wiederhold, Douglas P Gibson, Timothy Kimbrell, Teresa L Kramer, et al. "Heart Rate Variability and Cognitive Bias Feedback Interventions to Prevent Post-Deployment PTSD: Results from a Randomized Controlled Trial." *Military Medicine* 184, no. 1–2 (January 1, 2019): e124–32. https://doi.org/10.1093/milmed/usy171.

11. Feinstein, Justin S., Sahib S. Khalsa, Hung-wen Yeh, Colleen Wohlrab, W. Kyle Simmons, Murray B. Stein, and Martin P. Paulus. "Examining the Short-Term Anxiolytic and Anti-depressant Effect of Floatation-REST." *PLOS ONE* 13, no. 2 (February 2, 2018): e0190292. https://doi.org/10.1371/journal.pone.0190292.

12. Al Zoubi, Obada, Masaya Misaki, Jerzy Bodurka, Rayus Kuplicki, Colleen Wohlrab, William A. Schoenhals, Hazem H. Refai, et al. "Taking the Body off the Mind: Decreased Functional Connectivity between Somatomotor and Default-Mode Networks Following Floatation-REST." *Human Brain Mapping* 42, no. 10 (July 1, 2021): 3216–27. https://doi.org/10.1002/hbm.25429.

Chapter 11

1. Rubik, Beverly. "The Biofield Hypothesis: Its Biophysical Basis and Role in Medicine." *The Journal of Alternative & Complementary Medicine* 8, no. 6 (2002): 703–17.

2. George, Mark S., Ziad Nahas, Monica Molloy, Andrew M. Speer, Nicholas C. Oliver, Xing-Bao Li, George W. Arana, S. Craig Risch, and James C. Ballenger. "A Controlled Trial of

Daily Left Prefrontal Cortex TMS for Treating Depression."
Biological Psychiatry 48, no. 10 (November 15, 2000): 962–
70. https://doi.org/10.1016/S0006-3223(00)01048-9.

3. Davidson, Richard J., and William Irwin. "The Functional
Neuroanatomy of Emotion and Affective Style." *Trends in
Cognitive Sciences* 3, no. 1 (January 1, 1999): 11–21.
https://doi.org/10.1016/S1364-6613(98)01265-0.

4. Goleman, Daniel. *Destructive Emotions: How Can We
Overcome Them?: A Scientific Dialogue with the Dalai Lama.*
Bantam, 2004.

5. Nature As Last Resort: Qigong & How it's Used to Combat Fatal
Illness; An Interview with Doctor Pang Heming. *Heaven Earth:
The Chinese Art of Living*; Jan 1992. Volume1; Number 3.

6. Nature As Last Resort: Qigong & How it's Used to Combat Fatal
Illness; An Interview with Doctor Pang Heming. *Heaven Earth:
The Chinese Art of Living*; Jan 1992. Volume1; Number 3.

7. Bensimon, Moshe, Dorit Amir, and Yuval Wolf. "Drumming
through Trauma: Music Therapy with Posttraumatic Soldiers."
The Arts in Psychotherapy 35, no. 1 (January 1, 2008): 34–48.
https://doi.org/10.1016/j.aip.2007.09.002.

8. Stone, Bessel A. van der Kolk Laura, Jennifer West, Alison
Rhodes, David Emerson, Michael Suvak, and Joseph Spin-
azzola. "Yoga as an Adjunctive Treatment for Posttraumatic
Stress Disorder: A Randomized Controlled Trial." *The Journal
of Clinical Psychiatry* 75, no. 6 (June 27, 2014): 22573.
https://doi.org/10.4088/JCP.13m08561.

9. Harris, David Alan. "Dance/Movement Therapy Approaches to
Fostering Resilience and Recovery among African Adolescent

Torture Survivors." *Torture: Quarterly Journal on Rehabilitation of Torture Victims and Prevention of Torture* 17, no. 2 (2007): 134–55. PMID: 17728491

Chapter 12

1. Boyce, Richard, Sylvain Williams, and Antoine Adamantidis. "REM Sleep and Memory." *Neurobiology of Sleep* 44 (June 1, 2017): 167–77. https://doi.org/10.1016/j.conb.2017.05.001.
2. R. Stickgold, "Of Sleep, Memories and Trauma," Nature Neuroscience 10, no. 5 (2007): 540–42.
3. Burk, Larry. "Warning Dreams Preceding the Diagnosis of Breast Cancer: A Survey of the Most Important Characteristics." *EXPLORE* 11, no. 3 (May 1, 2015): 193–98. https://doi.org/10.1016/j.explore.2015.02.008.
4. Burk, Larry, DelMarie Wehner, and Mary Scott Soo. "Dreams Prior to Biopsy for Suspected Breast Cancer: A Preliminary Survey." *EXPLORE* 16, no. 6 (November 1, 2020): 407–9. https://doi.org/10.1016/j.explore.2020.03.002.
5. Sigerist HE. "A History of Medicine Volume 2: Early Greek, Hindu, and Persian Medicine." 1st ed. New York: Oxford University Press; 1987;63.
6. Griffiths, Roland R, Matthew W Johnson, Michael A Carducci, Annie Umbricht, William A Richards, Brian D Richards, Mary P Cosimano, and Margaret A Klinedinst. "Psilocybin Produces Substantial and Sustained Decreases in Depression and Anxiety in Patients with Life-Threatening Cancer: A Randomized Double-Blind Trial." *Journal of Psychopharmacology* 30, no.

12 (December 1, 2016): 1181–97.
https://doi.org/10.1177/0269881116675513.

7. Jerome, Lisa, Allison A. Feduccia, Julie B. Wang, Scott Hamilton, Berra Yazar-Klosinski, Amy Emerson, Michael C. Mithoefer, and Rick Doblin. "Long-Term Follow-up Outcomes of MDMA-Assisted Psychotherapy for Treatment of PTSD: A Longitudinal Pooled Analysis of Six Phase 2 Trials." *Psychopharmacology* 237, no. 8 (August 1, 2020): 2485–97. https://doi.org/10.1007/s00213-020-05548-2.

8. Feder, Adriana, Sarah B. Rutter, Daniela Schiller, and Dennis S. Charney. "Chapter Nine - The Emergence of Ketamine as a Novel Treatment for Posttraumatic Stress Disorder." In *Advances in Pharmacology*, edited by Ronald S. Duman and John H. Krystal, 89:261–86. Academic Press, 2020. https://doi.org/10.1016/bs.apha.2020.05.004.

9. Abdallah, Chadi G., Gerard Sanacora, Ronald S. Duman, and John H. Krystal. "The Neurobiology of Depression, Ketamine and Rapid-Acting Antidepressants: Is It Glutamate Inhibition or Activation?" *Pharmacology & Therapeutics* 190 (October 1, 2018): 148–58. https://doi.org/10.1016/j.pharmthera.2018.05.010.

10. Kennedy, David O., Wendy Little, and Andrew B. Scholey. "Attenuation of Laboratory-Induced Stress in Humans After Acute Administration of Melissa Officinalis (Lemon Balm)." *Psychosomatic Medicine* 66, no. 4 (2004). https://doi.org/10.1097/01.psy.0000132877.72833.71.

11. Kennedy, David O., Wendy Little, and Andrew B. Scholey. "Attenuation of Laboratory-Induced Stress in Humans After

Acute Administration of Melissa Officinalis (Lemon Balm)." *Psychosomatic Medicine* 66, no. 4 (2004). https://doi.org/10.1097/01.psy.0000132877.72833.71.

12. Rabinak, Christine A., Mike Angstadt, Maryssa Lyons, Shoko Mori, Mohammed R. Milad, Israel Liberzon, and K. Luan Phan. "Cannabinoid Modulation of Prefrontal–Limbic Activation during Fear Extinction Learning and Recall in Humans." *Extinction* 113 (September 1, 2014): 125–34. https://doi.org/10.1016/j.nlm.2013.09.009.

13. Van der Kolk, Bessel. "The Body Keeps the Score: Brain, Mind, and Body in the Healing of Trauma." *New York*, 2014.

INDEX

Index

assessing, 86
Heart and, 73, 74, 76, 86,
    96, 129, 133, 206
nature of, 73
trauma and, 96
Siegel, Bernie S., 44
silent meditation retreats, 48–
    51
sleep, 171–73
    REM, 171, 172, 178–79
    See also dreaming
small bowel obstruction
    (SBO), living with,
    21–22
Somatic Experiencing (SE),
    156–58
    deactivating trauma with,
        161–63
somatic therapies, 108. *See
    also specific topics*
Soubirous, Bernadette, 201–2
soul loss and soul retrieval,
    193–95
spirituality
    psychedelic-assisted, 183–
        86
    See also prayer; *specific
        topics*
Spleen energetic (TCM), 87,
    89–92
states vs. traits, 57–58
stress
    chronic, 13–14
    trauma and, 13, 17–18 (*see
        also* posttraumatic
        stress disorder)
    See also worry
subconscious awareness. *See*
    gut-brain; intuition
subpersonalities, 74–76. *See
    also* Parts Work

suffering and finding
    meaning, 114. *See
    also* Frankl, Viktor E.
Sullivan, Andrew, 48–50
superconscious awareness,
    72–74
    treatment and, 133–35,
        138, 139
    See also Heart-mind; near-
        death experiences
surgery without anesthesia,
    infant, 27
survivor guilt, 82–85

Temoshok, Lydia, 62
theater, trauma-informed, 164
traditional Chinese medicine
    (TCM), 102–3, 161
    emotions and, 85, 88–96
    Five-Element Theory, 72–
        74, 86–94, 94t
    sleep and, 173
    See also specific topics
traits vs. states, 57–58
transgenerational epigenetic
    inheritance, 35–36,
    116
trauma, 1, 2, 14–15, 209–11
    cancer and, 113, 210
    categories of therapies for,
        108
    definitions, 2, 14, 23–24,
        191 (*see also*
        wound that isn't
        healing)
    developmental, 26–31
    DSM and, 18, 20, 23
    nature of, 13, 23
    outcomes after, 18
    See also posttraumatic
        stress disorder;
        specific topics

Made in the USA
Middletown, DE
08 February 2025

71011972R00154